A Guide for Practitioners and Self-Cultivators

Cultivating The Thirteen Ghost Points

Clearing and Transcending Life's Traumas

By
Leta Herman
&
Jaye McElroy

Born Perfect® ink
Ancient Wisdom for Modern Times
Northampton, USA

www.BornPerfectInk.com
www.AlchemyLearningCenter.com

Cultivating The Thirteen Ghost Points: Clearing and Transcending Life's Traumas – A Guide for Practitioners and Self-Cultivators

FIRST EDITION, First Printing, May 2025

Cover Photo and Design: Jaye McElroy
Back Cover Photo and Design: Jaye McElory and Leta Herman
Photos in text: Jaye McElroy and Leta Herman

Editors: Leta Herman, Jaye McElroy, Jane Karras, Rosie Pearson, and Jennifer Abbingsole

Born Perfect®
17 New South St., Suite 108
Northampton, MA 01060, USA BornPerfectInk.com

Published in the United States of America by Born Perfect® ISBN: 979-8-9881971-2-6 (hard cover).

Important: The information and techniques discussed in this book are based upon the personal and professional experiences and research of its authors. The information contained in this book is not meant to be a substitute for medical care by a physician or other healthcare provider(s). Any diagnosis or medical care should be done under the guidance of a healthcare professional. The publisher does not promote the use of specific healthcare protocols but believes the information in this book should be made available to the general public. Neither the authors nor the publisher assume any liability whatsoever for the use of the information contained in this book. The authors and publisher strongly suggest consulting a professional healthcare provider about the appropriateness of any technique or procedure mentioned in this book.

Contents

Acknowledgments

We owe our deepest gratitude to every person who helped breathe life, wisdom, love, and deep compassion into this book, especially to our clients and students who've graced us with their presence, stories, and healing journeys throughout the years. Thank you.

As people who aren't originally from the Chinese Daoist culture (at least in this lifetime), we want to acknowledge with deep gratitude all those teachers (living and ancestral) who have generously shared their gifts with us. Our heartfelt love and appreciation goes to Master Jeffrey Yuen, an 88th generation Daoist priest, who's been our North Star, guiding us to explore our own self-cultivation and always encouraging us to seek more on this incredible journey of turning knowledge into experiential wisdom. For over two decades, we've actively absorbed and applied this body of knowledge, infusing it with our unique insights and experience. Our intention, as students of Daoism and Alchemy, is to responsibly and conscientiously carry this wisdom forward in a way that honors the lineages and the mentors who have influenced us and then share it as widely as possible for the betterment of all who may seek it.

We also want to express our deep appreciation for all the amazing people who have embarked on the path of Alchemy with us. Diving into the mystery of life takes courage and a deep sense of self-worth, self-love, and a dedication to self-cultivation. We're genuinely humbled to serve as companions and guides along their journeys. Being witness to the many incredible daily, weekly, monthly, and yearly personal changes, transformations, and experiences of spiritual growth is a gift we cherish. It truly inspires us every day.

We hope that each reader of this book finds it helpful along their own unique path of transformation. And we always like to add a little love and laughter in our lives along the way, which we think can work wonders on the healing journey! Our goal is to facilitate greater open-hearted authenticity in every facet of life for everyone and anyone seeking it.

All emotional ghosts
have a mortal fear.

All of this ancient formula
presented here!

Thirteen Points and they
disappear!

—**Sun SiMiao**
Ode of the Thirteen Ghost Points
Translator unknown

Preface

As some of the hidden gems of the acupuncture world, the Ghost Points are shrouded in mystery and often misunderstood. Even though the Ghost Points are largely ignored in modern-day Chinese Medicine, we believe that their transformational power is more relevant than ever in our current era.

One reason the Ghost Points generally don't receive much emphasis in modern Chinese Medicine practices is because they require practitioners to cultivate a deep understanding of themselves, and of these points as well, in order to effectively harness the wisdom of their transformative power and unlock their full potential. Cultivating the Thirteen Ghost Points goes beyond theoretical knowledge; it involves hands-on clinical experience in which the points become the instructive mentors. It's through observing the impact these points have on ourselves and our clients that their mysterious essence begins to be revealed.

The Thirteen Ghost Points are surprisingly relevant and extremely useful in modern-day Chinese Medicine practices. But before we talk about using them in today's modern clinical setting, let's go on a journey back in time...

Throughout history, well-known Chinese Medicine practitioners, such as Ge Hong, Sun SiMiao, and Ma Dan-Yang created a number of amazing and unique protocols to help unblock and free up our lives on these three levels: the body, the mind, and the spirit.

There are a few more legendary Daoist figures and doctors who we feel are important to mention, including Bian Que, Lu Dong Bin, and Sun Bu'Er (Ma Dan-Yang's brilliant wife), who have contributed to our knowledge and to the ever-deepening conversations about Chinese Medicine and Alchemy. These techniques and the resulting accumulation of knowledge have been passed down for generations and have come to us through a number of teachers, with the primary influence coming from the extraordinary Master Jeffrey Yuen, an 88th generation Daoist Priest.

The Ghost Points, originally a set of 20 points, were identified by a doctor named Bian Que, who was known as an almost mythical being who lived in the Warring States period (407–310 BCE). He was the earliest recorded Chinese doctor and likely a shaman, often pictured in a bird-like robe. Much later in history, a subset of his points were compiled by Sun SiMiao (581–682 CE) into the treatment protocol we know today as the Thirteen Ghost Points. This treatment has been used for many centuries to assist people navigating various levels of stuckness and "dis-ease," whether it's physical pain, emotional ruts, mental illness, or a severe trauma history.

As we delve into the exploration of these points, our intention with this book is to support our readers in navigating their own life's challenges, reshaping their personal narratives, reigniting their passion, and tapping into their own inherent magic and the magic of Alchemical Chinese Medicine. Additionally, we envision this book serving as a comprehensive guide and springboard for practitioners who are eager to understand, cultivate, and incorporate the Ghost Points into their practice.

While we strongly advocate for hands-on clinical mentorship for practitioners, we've reached a stage in our teaching where we believe that a written text can offer a meaningful level of understanding and can facilitate the widespread sharing of this knowledge among both practitioners and self-cultivators. Our aim is to make this work available to a much wider audience, extending its reach far beyond our personal capacity and putting it into the hands of potential students throughout the world.

What is Self-Cultivation?

The underlying concept of self-cultivation is to think of ourselves as gardeners, wherein the garden we tend is our inner landscape.

What kind of gardener are you? Are you a hands-off gardener who enjoys allowing natural plants to grow wherever they choose of their own accord? Or are you a cultivator... one who loves to plant and weed, creating an impeccably manicured garden? Or are you somewhere in between?

Self-cultivation is applying your consciousness to your inner garden realm. Even a hands-off gardener is consciously gardening, essentially meaning that they are cultivating wild gardens on purpose. This requires effort, as does the path of the impeccable gardener.

When you cultivate a garden, you must make some level of decision about where it will be dug and what will grow in it. When you cultivate yourself, it means that you make decisions about how you want to engage with your inner and outer life. Do you want to meditate? Do you want to go for long walks in nature? What are you thinking about? Who do you think you are? Do you believe you have a purpose in life and, if so, do you have awareness about whether your actions are leading you to that purpose? Do you have a sense of fulfillment in your day-to-day life that assures you that you are on that path? Do you hang onto past pain and hurts, and if so, are you aware of their influence on your life? These are just a few of the questions that self-cultivators might ask themselves, as they strive to discern which thoughts need to be weeded out and which truly reflect their authentic selves.

The type and amount of effort put into self-cultivation is extremely specific to the person doing the self-cultivating. It may include meditation or chanting or a tai chi or yoga practice, for example. It may include reading spiritual scriptures, communing with nature, observing the seasons, cultivating gratitude, or as simple as being truly kind to yourself. It may include many other possibilities. But in the efforts applied, the person feels a deeper sense of connection with their innermost self and the universe or the Dao.

> "The Dao that can be told is not the eternal Dao; The name that can be named is not the eternal name."
>
> **– Lao Tzu**

In this book, we use the term "self-cultivator" to refer to those who engage in this profound work for their own growth, rather than soley as practitioners treating others. We also believe that even practitioners must also be self-cultivators to fully harness the power of Alchemical Chinese Medicine in their practices.

While we emphasize the self-cultivation of the Ghost Points, we also want to highlight the significant advantage of receiving a Ghost Points treatment in person from a practitioner. As we explain later in the book, the Heart needs to speak, and the practitioner acts as a witness, making the entire experience quite magical.

A Note from Leta

I grew up in a culture that viewed the human body as a finely tuned machine, and modern science and Western medicine were revered as the way to address any bodily malfunction. If you fell ill, modern medicine would simply offer a pill to heal you. If you were injured, surgical procedures could put you back together. Magic and miracles had no place in this paradigm—there were only cold, hard facts and a few well-placed stitches to put you back together again if you needed them. Yet, for me, these cold, hard facts often contradicted each other, leaving me puzzled about the best path to health.

One year, the media hailed tofu as a superfood; the next year, soy was vilified for its estrogenic overloading properties. Eggs, too, experienced a rollercoaster ride of reputation, initially lauded for their health benefits, then demonized shortly thereafter, and ultimately reinstated as nutritional powerhouses only to still be questioned to this day for their validity in the healthy food category. Similarly, butter was ousted by margarine, only to reclaim its status as a dietary superstar by the popular Ketogenic and Paleo diets. While the much hailed Mediterranean diet encourages swapping butter out for olive oil, even that diet is also possibly on the chopping block as far as being a healthy choice! While exercise was universally touted as essential for well-being, cautionary tales emerged about the dangers of overexertion. Smoking tobacco, once depicted as a stress-reliever, faced a stark reversal when its association with fatal consequences became undeniable. The cycle of contradictory information seemed (and still seems) unending.

My beloved grandmother fell victim to the influence of the media. Battling obesity and diabetes, she cut back on sugar and embraced saccharine, which was, at the time, heralded as the best sugar substitute for weight loss. But then, suddenly, the tides turned, and a study came out saying that saccharine could potentially cause cancer. Shortly thereafter, she was given a devastating blow: a pancreatic cancer diagnosis. She soon passed away, convinced her illness stemmed from consuming too much saccharine.

Despite witnessing these contradictions in modern-day thinking, I still clung to the belief that the body was a machine that we could somehow maintain with pills and replacement parts if we only understood it better. Yet, somewhere within me, I sensed there was more to the story than what modern science was offering.

As a young child, I was drawn to nature, where I cultivated a love for plants and felt an almost mystical connection with them. I spent endless days outdoors, scaling trees, perching amidst their branches, talking to the birds, insects, and even the trees themselves. However, as I grew older, my experiences in nature seemed to clash with my evolving worldview, and gradually I began to forget about this intimate connection I'd had with the natural world.

Years later, when I was working in the tech industry in the Silicon Valley, a friend mentioned Plant Spirit Medicine teacher Eliot Cowan and handed me his book. I was at first skeptical, but the book jogged my memory of my love of plants as a child, bringing me to tears. It took me back to those young years and my connection with plants.

I was also pretty frustrated with modern medicine at the time. I had been in much pain for a number of years due to endometriosis. I believed surgery would heal me, but a few months after the operation, the pain returned. My doctor's response? She said, "Oh dear, we usually don't see the pain return for at least a year." I was shocked and saddened that I'd undergone surgery for, at best, a year's relief. Needless to say, I was desperate to find a new approach to healing.

Something deep down inside me pulled me towards Cowan's work. I enrolled in his training, undergoing a profound transformation that changed me from a logic-based systems engineer into a shamanic healer—a radical transition that didn't happen overnight but evolved over the next several years. In fact, I found Cowan's teachings very challenging intellectually and emotionally, especially the study of possession—the notion that entities or spirits could take people over, fully or partially. From a scientific standpoint, I had no framework for the idea of ghosts or a multidimensional, shamanistic paradigm. This concept clashed with everything I thought I knew, but, for some reason, I let the teachings from Cowan (and the teachings passed down from his teacher J.R.

Worsley and the Five Element Chinese Medicine tradition) enter deeply into my stream of consciousness.

Initially, I tried to rationalize the idea of possession as simply being another term for mental illness. That seemed to work for a while. However, after witnessing many unexplained phenomena in the treatment room, I became weary of this ever-thinning theory of mine. There was no way to explain what I was actually seeing, experiencing, and feeling within a scientific mindset.

I grappled with trepidation and nervousness as I started my own clinical practice and encountered clients in need of this work. There were so many questions: What were these "ghosts" in people? Were they like the ghosts in the movies? Were they friendly, like Casper the Friendly Ghost, or malevolent, vengeful spirits? The scariest movie I knew as a kid was *The Exorcist*, but how did real-life ghosts manifest? What is a true possession? Where do ghosts come from? And certainly I pondered whether they could be a danger to me or to those around me.

I later realized that such questions are normal for any practitioner entering this realm. Though the work was far from conventional, it felt totally right for me. It challenged me intellectually, emotionally, physically, and spiritually, sparking a sense of fascination and curiosity. It was new, exciting, and interesting every day. It still is! And to this day, I feel happy, fulfilled, and excited to do this work.

Gradually, I recognized that the body was more than a mere machine and that healing transcended mechanical fixes. Healing, in its essence, was magical and exhilarating. The phrase "mind blown" became my frequent daily companion during this journey.

Fortunately, a mentor appeared in my life: Niki Bilton, former Dean at J.R. Worsley's college. I immersed myself in her clinic and classroom, seeking answers to my lingering questions. I craved guidance, and soaked up every last bit of clinical wisdom she was offering. If there is one thing about me, it's my insatiable curiosity to know more and to dig deeper into the mysteries of this work.

I began attending her healing intensives on possession treatments. The rigorous schedule consisted of seven consecutive days, nearly 24 hours a day. It pushed me to my limits. It was like being thrown into the deep end of the pool to learn how to swim... and no swimmies on your arms to keep you afloat!

Initially focused on Worsley-style treatments, Bilton later introduced Sun SiMiao's Thirteen Ghost Points to our group of students. Bilton held the belief that all the points should be done in a single session, without time constraints—an approach I later learned is not typical in modern practices. This method, essential to our training, meant that treatments could extend anywhere from four to twelve hours, adapting to the client's individual rhythm and the practitioner's level of expertise and self-cultivation.

In 2004, I had the opportunity to attend a lecture by Master Jeffrey Yuen at the New England School of Acupuncture in Boston with Bilton and a number of her students. The lecture focused on Alchemical Acupuncture and delved into the origins of the Thirteen Ghost Points, along with their practical application.

Attending the 2004 workshop was a turning point for me, because once I met Master Yuen, I knew that he was to be my life teacher. He was the huge missing piece in my Chinese Medicine learning puzzle that just effortlessly fell into place. I attended his two-year advanced Classical Chinese Medicine course in New York City starting in 2006 and have since been to China a number of times and traveled the world with him.

Master Yuen's emphasis on the magic of healing and Alchemical theories resonates deeply with me. I have seamlessly integrated his teachings with those of my past mentors, gradually evolving my own style and teaching approach.

Today, my teaching style is a fusion of Master Yuen's lecture-style teachings and Bilton's focus on clinical observation and supervision. Our Master Alchemy Apprenticeship Program (MAAP) embodies this fusion, offering both theoretical instruction and hands-on clinical observation and supervision with a huge focus on self-cultivation. It also emphasizes that advanced students learn to do the entire protocol with no time constraints, so that the healing can unfold organically.

In 2012, Jaye McElroy joined me in teaching this work, injecting it with her unique approach and intuition that is centered on self-discovery and self-cultivation for practitioner and layperson alike.

This was another piece of the puzzle that just made everything click, creating a beautiful synergy in our work together. While our work is rooted in Bilton's and Yuen's teachings, our approach heavily emphasizes self-cultivation, aiming to enrich each practitioner's own authenticity and growth. Together, we aim to breathe life into these points, not only as tools for treatments but also as allies in each individual's healing journey.

A Note from Jaye

When I first crossed paths with Leta shortly after the start of her Alchemical journey, it was as if a veil had been lifted, revealing Alchemy as my destined path. The language of the Five Elements resonated deeply with me and felt like something I'd instinctively known my whole life but never had the vocabulary to express.

Attending Master Yuen's lecture on the Nine Palaces of the Heart alongside Leta marked a pivotal moment in my journey as a marketing coach and life strategist. Immersing myself in all the literature I could find on the Five Elements, the Nine Palaces, and Alchemy, I felt like I'd found something I'd been seeking that I hadn't realized I was looking for.

As I began to witness the transformative power of the Ghost Points and other related Alchemy treatments, I realized that clients who'd undergone the Thirteen Ghost Points treatments exhibited a greater capacity to engage more deeply with the life strategies we developed together—empowering them to rewrite their narratives and embrace fresh perspectives. The Ghost Points, in particular, seemed to unlock a sense of freedom within my clients, allowing them the ability to make choices without self-judgment.

My role as a business/marketing coach underwent a remarkable transformation... into what I now call Alchemical Life Strategy work. Instead of navigating through layers of complexity with my clients, I found myself simply holding space and reflecting back the authentic selves my clients were aspiring to be. Our work together became a collaborative journey toward crafting their ideal lives. While obstacles still arose, the Ghost Points transformed what once seemed like an insurmountable tangle of threads into manageable challenges.

I wanted to share my perspective in this book as an initial bystander who admired Alchemy work, and then found a way to incorporate it into my work and my life, offering my version to others through support, encouragement, and strategic conversations, all rooted in an open heart, free from judgment.

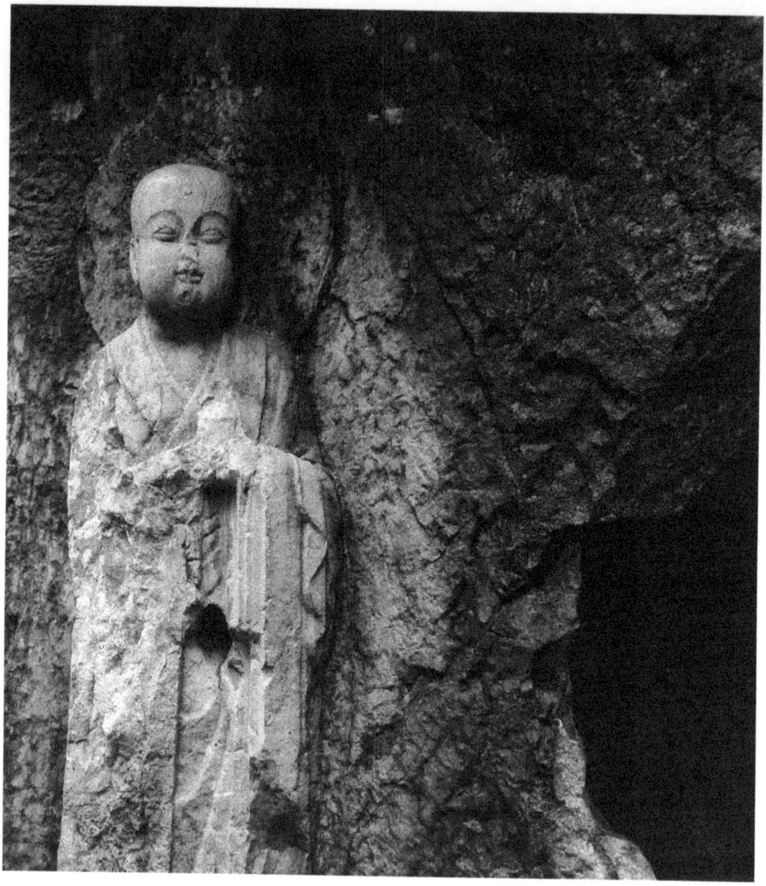

Guadian Monk from FeiLai Feng, Hangzhou, China

PART ONE: SELF-CULTIVATORS AND PRACTITIONERS ARE THE SAME

This section introduces you to the various ways you can utilize the Ghost Points in your life and in your practice. Whether you come to this work as a lay person interested in healing yourself or your loved ones, or you are already a practitioner, you will want to cultivate these points for yourself before working with others.

The Sage knows the world because whatever's happening outside is happening inside.

—Master Jeffrey Yuen

Chapter One: Why Can't You Just Be Yourself?

Deep down, we all crave the ability to embrace and love life with our arms wide open. It's a feeling of being so present and connected—as if we're plugged into the very essence of existence—a feeling many of us may recall from our earliest childhood days. Isn't that the essence of what we all want or seek?

Sadly, life doesn't always deliver love, excitement, happiness, and pure joy on a silver platter. As we go through life, we meet obstacles on our journey and feel thwarted. This is natural.

Instead of feeling alive in the moment, we might feel tangled up in feelings of fear, worry, disconnection, stress, sadness, or what we call *the boredom epidemic*. It's like being stuck in a pit of quicksand—a mire that's tough to break free from.

The reasons why we can end up in this stuck state are so numerous and so common that they are seemingly endless in supply. Sometimes, it's as simple as thinking that something or someone is blocking our path. It's the feeling of being stuck in a traffic jam that's not our fault.

Eventually (and hopefully) the traffic clears on its own, things shift, and life's obstacles seem to move to the side of the road or simply move out of sight. The moment the roadblock shifts, it can feel like a river's dam opening up, and then suddenly, we're back in the flow, riding down our own lifestream again—this time going in the right direction. Once we start flowing, it can feel exhilarating, motivating, and like a big sigh of relief, especially if we've been stuck for a long time.

The cycle of feeling stuck and then getting relief as we overcome obstacles is a universal human experience that we all encounter at various points in our lives.

But what if you feel like the traffic jam has no end in sight? What if you can't shake a bad birth story, a very difficult childhood, traumatic early life events, or even traumatic events carried over from a past life? What if you're unable to break free on your own or catch a glimpse of the open road? What if you're not just physically stuck, but emotionally and mentally stuck as well. It might feel like you're on autopilot, and just going through the motions.

In the worst cases, this feeling of being perpetually stuck can lead to some really dark places, like a heavy weight of despair from which there seems to be no escape.

If you've felt any of these states of being, you might just think these are the cards life dealt you and there's nothing you can do to change it. Even when the situation isn't that dire... even when it's more about the daily grind and just going through the motions, it can still be incredibly challenging if you feel like you can't seem to get any traction. It may wear you down, even causing you to lower your expectations of happiness and joy to the point that you've lost hope.

We believe that this doesn't have to be the case. In fact, we've seen enough examples to know that life doesn't have to be hard or full of struggles... at all! Let's explore another viewpoint—a paradigm shift that could truly set you free from past baggage or trauma. Could it really be easy to be happy in our lives, or what Jaye likes to call, *happy on the way to happiness*? You can change your life and yourself. You can find your way forward to your true self, your authentic nature.

State of Mind vs. State of Medicine

Modern-day medicine practices throughout most of the world are based on the idea that people contract a disease or experience an injury that causes them discomfort. To heal in the modern medicine paradigm, you simply need to take a pharmaceutical and the symptoms will disappear. End of story. No new behaviors are required, no looking into the cause (just the hoped-for effects), and almost zero time is spent on deep spiritual self-cultivation or overall wellness.

On top of this emphasis on healing coming from something outside of you, modern medicine often encourages you as the patient to comply with your doctor's instructions and ignore your own instincts, feelings, and thoughts. And while there are some doctors who are moving away from this belief system, most of them still seem to support it. Even if what the doctor suggests that you do (take some medicine or get this surgery) instinctively feels bad to you, you still feel that you should continue to override your inner awareness and do what the doctor says.

Alchemical Chinese Medicine disrupts the old paradigm of the "doctor knows best" and "patients are ignorant" roles. In fact, with Alchemy, the Alchemical practitioner takes the role of facilitator in the healing session, which means holding space for healing, not actually "helping" at all. Instead of a practitioner being "in charge," you, the patient, are in charge. Your practitioner trusts your destiny path, even to the point of accepting that your "illness" has arisen to provoke a change. Your practitioner is there simply to walk alongside you and encourage you to do what is necessary for the curriculum lessons of your lifetime.

With Alchemy, we shift away from modern-day medicine's focus on simple survival and "getting their patients back into the workforce as soon as possible," or what, for eons, used to be simply "hunting and gathering." Hunting and gathering in our modern world typically consists of going to work, coming home, consuming some form of sustenance, indulging in distractions of some kind, trying to sleep, and then getting up to go to work the next day—*rinse and repeat.*

If that's the goal—to not have to change anything that is causing the health crisis—then this type of medicine is going to be focused on only a handful of areas: digestion, breathing, movement, and sleeping. Whenever any of these basic functions of life aren't working, you *will* feel quite unwell. But this approach is only about surviving; it's not about thriving. We have accepted short-term-functional, unhealthy living as a new norm.

More and more, however, the issues that arise from modern forms of illness appear to be affecting our lives much more deeply than the day-to-day survival issues—both physically and psychologically. The more advanced our society becomes, the more psycho-spiritual illnesses we seem to see. It's as if the rise in anxiety and depression today ironically correlates to the relatively greater ease we now have in our daily lives. If we have more time to contemplate our lives because we're not working so hard to survive day-to-day (literal hunting and gathering), that means we have more time to focus on the psycho-spiritual struggles that stem from obsessive thinking. In other words, obsessive thinking seems to increase when we have more spare time to do it.

In Alchemical Chinese Medicine, the Ghost Points are one of the most effective tools for breaking free from the obsessive-thinking loop. Worry, anxiety, and depression are all different expressions of obsessive thinking. These feelings can stem from a variety of sources, such as childhood abuse, toxic relationships, bullying, a sense of not belonging, and many other factors.

The idea behind all of these negative experiences is that they hook into the psyche and become embedded, and we can't let them go. We are like a fish on a hook, and it's very difficult to get free. We even have new names for illnesses and completely new syndromes and diseases that we've never seen before. These involve severe systemic dysfunction and are often thought to be connected to psychological or emotional issues. Even modern medicine is beginning to acknowledge the link between emotional issues and a person's health, as with autoimmune diseases, gastrointestinal illness, cardiovascular disease, high blood pressure, and many other physical disorders as well as mental ones. Also, in this post-COVID era, with climate change and the worries and fears about increasing violence, many new reports show that citizens of the modern world are facing multiple and compounded major mental health emergencies.

The most glaring epidemic of all is loneliness, which of course became more prevalent during the COVID lockdown. We are clearly more connected to each other electronically than ever before, but we are also more separated physically than ever before. Younger people are losing the social skills and open-heartedness needed to connect with others in the physically present world, as opposed to online or via text, making it more difficult to have deeper relationships. In fact things have gotten so bad recently that in 2023, the US Surgeon General released a General Advisory on the Healing Effects of Social Connection and Community called: Our Epidemic of Loneliness and Isolation. In this report there are many alarming statistics pointing to our increasing loneliness, such as this statistic:

> *Approximately half of U.S. adults report experiencing loneliness, with some of the highest rates among young adults.*

The report also claims that social media use may be a factor:

> *In a U.S.-based study, participants who reported using social media for more than two hours a day had about double the odds of reporting increased perceptions of social isolation compared to those who used social media for less than 30 minutes per day.*

The World Health Organization estimates that 970 million people in the world suffer from mental or behavioral disorders, over 280 million have depression, and approximately 301 million have anxiety.[1] Close to 800,000 die from suicide every year, which is the forth leading cause of death for people ages 15 to 29.[2]

Why Alchemical Chinese Medicine is Different

Alchemical Chinese Medicine offers another perspective on healing. What if instead of focusing on *not being ill*, we turn towards the question: What would help us truly *thrive* in life?

Ancient Alchemical Chinese Medicine is focused on spiritual growth and transformation rather than simply returning you back to a previous state of being. The goal isn't to get you back to when you once felt good... the goal is to move you forward and beyond. A metamorphosis of change is often the result.

We can look at most modern physical and mental illness as challenges to our ability to live authentically according to our true nature or temperament. Sometimes a person's qi or energy becomes *inauthentic*. Someone or something is blocking qi flow. The person is no longer able to be free to choose their true path in life. The block could be a person, a place, a thing, or an emotional trauma from either this life, a past life, or something that has been passed down genetically from ancestors.

The magic of Alchemy helps you not just heal but transform—even transmute. We know that the use of words like magic, metamorphosis, transformation, and transmutation

---

[1] Mental Disorders Fact Sheet, World Health Organization, https://www.who.int/news-room/fact-sheets/detail/mental-disorders.

[2] Suicide Fact Sheet, World Health Organization, https://www.who.int/news-room/fact-sheets/detail/suicide.

may cause some people to roll their eyes and put this book down as a result—and we are okay with that! There will be others who will find this language motivating, inspiring, and hopeful! We are always hopeful that people can find a way to be open-minded and open-hearted to the possibility—and in fact, to *all possibilities*.

The transformative power of Thirteen Ghost Point treatments taps into the Alchemical principle of using healing to facilitate a larger self-actualization. More than just eliminating disease, Alchemy seeks to revive the vital spark within each patient to burn brighter. Thus, a single Ghost Point session holds the potential to radically shift not just symptoms, but a patient's entire life narrative.

These treatments are not about waving a magical wand or chanting an incantation, although both those things could happen in a Thirteen Ghost Points treatment. Nothing is beyond reason when it supports a person's transformation. These sessions are *a portal* to a healing journey for both the client and the practitioner, where old paradigms can fall away and unhelpful identity structures can dissolve as patients recognize more expansive truths about themselves and reality. The person's life force can dissolve energetic ice dams so that energy can begin flowing freely again. As a result the *magic* of the treatment arises from the person's willingness to change. What emerges then sparkles with new vitality.

Mainstream Chinese Medicine, as it's most commonly taught, utilizes the Primary Channel system (the meridian pathways in the body) for the necessary maintenance of life, attempting to keep the patient grounded and able to function in life. The Primary Channel system can also be mystical with points like the Source Points and the Back *Shu* (*Shu* means pivot, meaning transformational) points. This system often offers a slow evolutionary approach, one that can take many years, to help a person move forward along their path.

The Ghost Points treatment, on the other hand, can help restart and reorient the whole physiological system, accessing the deep matrices that hold old trauma patterns. Releasing these patterns then allows larger-scale psychological and spiritual shifts in a relatively short period of time.

We believe that the Ghost Points can help a person align with their natural rhythms so that their dormant inner potential can emerge, like a phoenix rising from the ashes of former limitations. It is a deeper awakening of what already lies within.

Thus, while Chinese Medicine traditionally fosters change through steady ongoing treatments, the Alchemical approach can spark quantum leaps in a short time period. Alchemy isn't just transformation... it's *transmutation.* Tranformation is evolutionary adaptation that inches along generation by generation, sometimes taking thousands of years to evolve. In contrast, Alchemy pursues radical transmutation within an individual's lifetime.

Imagine flipping your life 180 degrees. It's a little disorientating at first! So there has to be a period of adjustment with that level of change. This period can take one second, one day, three months, six months or even up to a year, depending on the person. There is no standard timeline, each person is different.

Alchemy and alchemical treatments can liberate us from whatever's restraining us, even if we don't know what that "thing" is. Alchemy can guide us to our authentic selves, shedding the baggage of not just this lifetime but even the burdens of our past lives or our ancestry.

This powerful healing work gives a person the chance to start with a clean slate and fresh possibilities. It promotes the authenticity of each person, releasing the habits of perception that were in place to provide protection. When we can break free from those old habits of perception and truly align with our authentic selves, everything just flows, and this allows for a profound metamorphosis. From this perspective, Alchemy becomes more than a healing modality—it becomes a spiritual path. We can unlock our full potential and learn how to spread our wings and soar.

Ghost Points Throughout History

The origins of the Ghost Points trace back to the first known, almost mythical Chinese physician, Bian Que (407–310 BCE), who actually created a total of twenty-one Ghost Points. Legend describes him as a magical being who could see through walls and even right into the human body. His healings were miraculous, and he even supposedly performed the very first heart transplant. In an ancient stone carving, he was actually depicted as a bird with a human head, though this may have been a shamanic bird headdress.

Moving forward in time, to around 1400 years ago, Sun SiMiao (581–682 CE) assembled thirteen of the twenty-one points into a protocol called the *Ode of the Thirteen Ghost Points*. Sun SiMiao is known as the King of Medicine in China, and most temples in China have statues or paintings of him on display. His work at that time built on the work of his contemporary, Chao Yuanfang, who wrote the *General Treatise on Causes and Manifestations of All Diseases*.

Sun SiMiao was an Alchemist and legend says he is an immortal. He believed that it was not necessary to take poisonous elixirs made out of minerals like mercury to achieve immortality (like his predecessor and mentor Ge Hong); rather you could cultivate yourself through acupuncture, herbal medicine, and meditation, or what's known as *Nei Dan* or Inner Alchemy.

He originally created the Ode of the Thirteen Ghost Points to cast out demons. The Ode was documented in his book called Essential Formulas for Emergencies Worth a Thousand Pieces of Gold. The demons were thought of as Ghosts, called *Gui* in Chinese. A Ghost is something outside of you that gets in and takes over, what we might call possession. Even an infestation of parasites can be seen as a possession.

Interestingly, however, this treatment wasn't meant to *only* address external factors. Humans are capable of creating their own mental demons, born from their inner thoughts and persistent fixations—what we might now label as our obsessions. We might call these the "Internal Causes of Disease" in Chinese Medicine.

The protocol isn't just a set of points that are meant to be used in any old order. In fact, they are in a very particular and quite ingenious order. The deeper we delve into this protocol, the more we appreciate the brilliance behind Sun SiMiao's selection of these thirteen points and the rationale for their specific order. In fact, we believe that *the Ghost Points possess a broader purpose beyond just dispelling inner and outer turmoil. They hold spiritual potential, not solely for banishing evil spirits, but also for nurturing inner cultivation and growth.*

What are Ghosts?

The term *Gui* or ghost, as we will be using it in our book, isn't necessarily a supernatural entity or even Casper the Friendly Ghost, as your mind might have conjured up, but rather something that's subverting your true essence in some way. More specifically, ghosts represent imprints left by past traumas, negative life experiences or relationships, or even just not fitting into your family or community.

When you undergo these negative experiences, the "ghosts" get hooked into you and generate suffering. The reason you get hooked in the first place is that you have an opening for the hook, in the way that a fish has to bite a hook in order to get caught. Something in you has invited the ghost to become hooked into you. And the Ghost Points provide an opportunity to regain freedom from the hooks we've taken in that are now holding us back from the authentic expression of our spirit and the authentic road we need to walk in life.

If you believe in life after death and the possibility of disembodied entities potentially possessing a human (which is part of the Chinese Medicine belief system), then "ghosts" could also be real ghosts, the way we normally think of them, either friendly or demonic. The Thirteen Ghost Points are also capable of "casting out demons," so to speak. And if you believe an entity can possess a person, then as a practitioner, you will be working with these "ghosts."

NOTE: The word *Gui* in Chinese refers only to the disembodied spirits that can possess people. But throughout this book, we will be using the word "ghosts" in quotation marks to signify that we are using the term more broadly than just referring to disembodied ghosts.

Part of the cultivation of the practitioner is to see these *Gui* as people too (even if they are non-physical). In this case, we have to learn to treat them as we would treat any other client.

If we look at the traditional types of ghosts (hungry, wandering, or romantic), we can see how this ancient information can be pertinent to our modern lives.

- The *hungry* ghost represents a ghost who constantly needs to consume. In today's modern world, it could relate to issues of overeating, obesity, shopping, hoarding, and addictions to such things as drugs, alcohol, information, or even social media.

- The *wandering* ghost represents a ghost who is feeling unsettled and looking around for something better all the time. It's associated with the need to travel, which means you don't feel happy where you currently are at any given moment. The *Gui* wants to have more experiences and stimulation, so it keeps you moving around. In modern life, it translates to the rise in anxiety and a feeling of dissatisfaction that might spur excessive use of media as a way to travel the world and see new things.

- The *romantic* ghost, also called the *sexual* ghost, was considered to be someone who dies but can't release an attachment to a loved one after death and continues to hang around as a ghost. It also could be related to feelings of lack of belonging, loneliness, or sexual addictions, such as a pornography addiction.

We believe it's not that important in modern times to know what kind of *Gui* a person has, but that it's more important to simply know that we have a tool in the Thirteen Ghost Points to make a significant change when a person is struggling.

The Ghost Points break through these obsessive infatuations, reaching into the core essence of the person, and allowing them access to their true selves. Whether the points are also "casting out demons" becomes a moot point. What matters isn't so much whether it's an entity or an obsessive thought form: What matters is finding freedom in yourself to be yourself.

What Does a *Gui* Look Like in a Person?

Can you think about a time when you've just met a person, and you get a nagging feeling that "something's not quite right?" Something is just off with them, but it's hard to put it into words. It's like there's a cloud veiling their true essence, hiding it deep beneath the surface.

As humans, we might not consciously be aware of someone's true nature, but many of us can sense when something is "off" about them. We can, however, hone the skill of discerning the authenticity of a person, gauging whether their true essence is being overshadowed by possession or obsession.

If you tend to be more clairvoyant, you might see it as a murky aura, like a gray cloud shrouding the person's countenance. If you're more clairsentient (someone who is tuned into feeling energy), you might feel something toxic lingering within them. For those who are more clairaudient (someone who hears psychic sounds or communications), you might perceive it as a dissonance or lack of authenticity in their voice. And for those who are claircognizant (someone who has a intuitive knowing), you might just receive information without the use of your senses at all.

The Magic of Alchemy

Alchemy isn't about the magical feats and sleight of hand of the greatest magicians throughout history. Alchemy is about the beauty, the mystery, and the magic of the heart and its ability to heal itself—sometimes instantaneously. During Alchemy treatments, we've witnessed the most incredible moments that were life-changing, dimensional-shifting, mind-bending events and sequences that one could never imagine or re-create. The experiences have been magical: random musical lyrics in sync with exactly what the client is saying at a given moment, candles burning in the room taking on a life of their own, even melting sideways, the walls of a room appearing to tilt on a side angle, even a sudden drop in temperature that defied explanation when there were no windows open, treatment room doors flying wide open for no apparent reason (although we believe everything happens for a reason), another being talking through a client with a completely different sounding voice... This list goes on and on.

These aren't just quirky events, although they certainly are quirky! They're part of the Alchemical journey of working with someone when you are working in the magical inner space we call "the void of the heart." Once we step into the magic of the heart, we're exploring other dimensions, sometimes bending the edges of reality, sometimes turning the ordinary into the extraordinary.

The Divine DJ of the Universe is At Your Command

The musical component of Alchemical treatments is one of the factors that make them truly amazing. Music has always been an integral part of Daoist ritual, including healing sessions. We believe that in ancient times, music played a key role in the Thirteen Ghost Points treatments. Monks, priests, or practitioners would participate in these treatments ritualistically, playing instruments and chanting. The movement of the treatment would often shift with the vibration of the music and the energy in the room.

While traveling in China, we got to personally witness one such ritual at the temple on top of the sacred Daoist mountain, Mao Shan. The priest was accompanied by ten other monks who played instruments and chanted throughout the ceremony to bless us—the travelers to the mountain and the temple. The music was an integral part of the magic of this hour-long ceremony that ebbed and flowed naturally—sometimes frenetic, sometimes ethereal, and sometimes emotionally moving. The music was so powerful, it brought tears to the eyes of some people who were present, including Jaye.

For many years now, we've tried to simulate or re-create this type of expression of improvisational music by using randomly shuffled playlists. We started with CD changers and iPods in the past and, over time, that has evolved into streaming playlists comprised of over 25,000 songs, inspirational and spiritual recordings, spoken word poetry, and stand-up comedy. We call this our "Divine DJ" because the music selections that arise during treatments often feel profound and magical and uniquely tailored to each person.

The Magic of Music

One of the stories Leta likes to recount took place during a treatment when a children's song called "Three is a Magic Number" came up randomly on her iPod, the device that replaced the CD changer and that she had used for years to create a magical music experience for her clients. The woman receiving treatment was trying to decide whether or not to have another baby. She had one child already and had lost her second baby. The song's refrain was, "A man and a woman had a little baby... they had three in the family, that's a magic number."

The woman asked right away, "Is that the answer to my question?" Leta did not know the answer to the question and simply stayed in the moment of the treatment. The client thought it seemed like too much of a coincidence, and she contemplated its relevance to her situation... until the next day. The woman returned for her follow-up treatment, which was in a different room with a different iPod and stereo system. As the treatment started, Leta pressed the shuffle button on the iPod, and much to their surprise, the exact same song, "Three is a Magic Number," came on again! It's as if the universe was conspiring to bring that song at the perfect moment. The sheer randomness of this is unthinkable to even try to understand, but it is something we see in the treatment room daily... nearly impossible coincidences that seem to validate the client's authentic experience in life.

A Shining Light Show

Another example of this type of synchronicity involved a young man struggling with anxiety and depression. During his Ghost Points treatment, he had been working on his traumatic experiences and limiting beliefs. As he was working through some difficult memories, things began to come to a head in the treatment. A long Van Morrison song (about nine minutes) came on, and as the song built momentum, lyrics about imminent change began to repeat themselves, over and over: "Change is coming, change is coming..." as if the song was responding to his anguish. These lyrics came at the very moment when he was facing how stuck he'd been feeling about his situation, perfectly mirroring the very palpable sense of the treatment coming to a climax.

At that precise moment, the song suddenly shifted too, with new lyrics: "I'm going to walk down the street to find my shining light." At the same time, a dimmable light fixture in the room inexplicably began to flicker through all its settings (there were three) over and over again as the shining light lyrics were repeated many times. The treatment just continued along as we were essentially being treated to a light and music show of the Divine DJ.

In hindsight, this was a pivotal moment for my client as he recognized the miraculousness of what he had witnessed that day. From that point on, his life turned around. Over time, his depression lifted and then cleared. He began to courageously pursue his passions and felt much more accepted by his family and peers. He found his inner connection and began to see the good inside himself.

Was there a spiritual connection between the musical synchronicity of the lyrics/light show and his transformation? We can't know for sure. However, for him, it validated something within him that continued to unfold after the treatment. For him, the song lyrics and the flickering light mirrored and solidified the awakening he felt after working through his block. This gave him permission at a deep level to forge ahead into his life with access to his full potential.

Ancestral Visitations from Parents

In one session, the client seemed to be a bit skeptical about the ability to shift some of her pain. But after about an hour, the magic of the Divine DJ shifted everything. A song from Phantom of the Opera soundrack came on, singing her name over and over. Suddenly, she started to understand the song as a message from her deceased mother and everything in the treatment turned around. She completely opened up and the real work of healing the pain in her heart began.

The following is a story from another one of our clients about his experience with the Divine DJ in an Alchemy treatment:

"When we came to the last point, I immediately knew what song came on... it was the slow movement from Dvorák's symphony, *From the New World*. My parents, who passed away over a decade ago, were classical musicians and probably would have played that piece multiple times with the symphony orchestra. I grew up with this music, and I know it really well. I was surprised it was on the playlist, because it had only been pop and hip-hop style music up until then. Suddenly the door to the treatment room just opened by itself. There was no draft in the room, and I don't even remember it being windy that day. The music swelled, and I could feel my parents coming to either side of me, laying their heads on my shoulders. I just felt total peace, and everything was okay. Nothing needed to happen. There was nothing to do. The music went from gentle and beautiful to spry and energetic. We listened to the whole movement—probably like eight or nine minutes long. I leaked gentle tears and cherished that visit I had with my parents.

"I wouldn't really say that I was actively grieving my parents like I would have after their passing. This was more like a visitation from them and an experience of entering into the realm of ancestors. It was a really timeless experience."

Magic Can Work in Mysterious Ways

The magical power of these Alchemical treatments can manifest in so many ways beyond music. It can appear in light, sound, air flow, nature, and pretty much anything you can imagine.

Mother May I?

We wrote about this treatment session in our book, *Through the Mystery Gate*, but it was a unique one and we wanted to include it here as well! Many years ago, a client brought her mother along to her all-day Ghost Point treatment, and she requested that her mother wait in the waiting room. We generally do not recommend that someone (especially your mother!) come to a Ghost Point treatment and wait in the waiting room because you often need to feel like you can speak freely without worrying about anyone else overhearing. But our clinic at the time was in a rural area and this woman had driven a very long distance. So of course we invited her mother to wait in the waiting room.

As the treatment progressed over the next few hours, the treatment room door repeatedly flew open, revealing her mother sitting on the waiting room couch, reading a book. Each time the door swung open, the mother jumped up to close the door, never saying a word. Although the story before this one referred to a door opening by itself, it had never happened before in any previous sessions in this building... ever!

It felt like a cosmic nudge to explore this further, leading us to dig a little deeper into her childhood and her relationship with her mother. The client suddenly remembered her mother telling her about how as an infant, she incessantly cried and that her colic had profoundly distressed her mother at the time. If that door had not magically swung open several times, reminding her about her mother out in the waiting room, we might never have uncovered this story or been able to bring closure and healing to both women. After that session, the client's extreme, mysterious, and sometimes debilitating anxieties completely vanished—one hundred percent.

The Silent Snow Squall Show

Not all Alchemical treatments must have music. The Divine can work with all kinds of aspects of the environment surrounding the treatment. In one session, the person requested no music due to her extreme sensitivities to sound. Leta agreed, with the understanding that the musical Divine DJ would be playing with the sound turned off and the lyrics displayed on a large screen instead. In this treatment, a few of our student apprentices were attending, and they could see the lyrics.

The lyrics were a powerful yet silent musical contribution to the long treatment. But the thing that really made the biggest impact did not come from the music but from the atmosphere surrounding the treatment. At one point, everything seemed to slow down, and we shared the silence and stillness of the room together, looking deeply into each others' eyes. The treatment room overlooked a big valley with mountain peaks behind it. Suddenly, outside, a whirlwind of snow came from out of nowhere. The entire sky was filled with falling snow—a complete whiteout. It was perfect for the client. The snow, which had not been forecasted and was completely unexpected, was symbolic for her, and the entire treatment shifted at that moment.

Where the Extraordinary Becomes Ordinary

When you step into the magic of Alchemical healing, you may likely experience similar remarkable moments that will leave you awestruck... on a daily basis! This becomes a journey into the extraordinary and profound. It's about being open to the mystical, embracing it, and realizing that the impossible can, in fact, become a reality. You just cannot predict or expect anything to go as planned or to be predictable once it starts!

One key factor of these treatments is for the practitioner to remain open-minded with no expectations about what they think may or may not happen. The practitioner isn't there to "fix" the person, but rather to be a facilitator walking the path through the points with that person, holding that sacred space in that very present moment in time. This is a radical new way to look at treatments in a modern day healing practice.

As you delve into the realm of the Ghost Points, you'll experience them not simply as acupuncture points on the body but as conduits into the mystical, unlocking inner potential, and connecting with the very essence of life. One big question you can ask yourself as either a practitioner, a client, or a self-cultivator of Alchemy: Are you ready to step into this world of wonder to become a part of the magical tapestry that is Alchemy? If your answer is yes, then welcome aboard! Your unique journey awaits, and it could be the most amazing and transformational experience of your life!

In nature there is no alienation

Everything belongs...

Our alienation is self-generated.[3]

—Deng Ming-Dao

---

[3] Deng Ming-Dao, 365 *Tao: Daily Meditations* New York: HarperOne, 1992),

Chapter Two: Where to Start? Right Here!

Whether you are a practitioner aiming to work with these points on others, or you're a self-cultivator wanting to learn the secrets of the Ghost Points for your own transformation, in both cases, it's essential to first cultivate these points within yourself. In fact, we see self-cultivation as a lifelong practice required to stay on the Alchemical path.

In this chapter, we'll discuss some foundational concepts necessary for your self-cultivation journey. Practitioners might find this a review, but given the vastness of Chinese Medicine, it's beneficial to revisit these key ideas together to enhance your development as a potential Ghost Points practitioner.

The Two Phases of Alchemy

So let's begin with a discussion about the approaches we use in Alchemy to help us realign with our true qi while embracing our own personal growth along the way.

There are two phases of Alchemy:

Clearing: First we focus on clearing a person's "ghosts" (or our own ghosts if we're self-cultivating) and getting the true qi flowing again in order to manifest the true essence of who we are.

Transforming: The second phase is consciously walking the path of Alchemy and moving forward through deep transformational stages, which in this book we call the *Nine Stages of Alchemy.*

This book will only focus on the first phase—the clearing aspect—which is the function of the Thirteen Ghost Points. To read more about the second phase, please read our previous book, *Through the Mystery Gate*, which explains all of the Nine Stages of Alchemy in more detail.

Clearing the Energy Blocks that Block Us

What is an energy block? An energy block is something that hinders the smooth flow of your vital life force (qi) through your body. Imagine a traffic jam with cars backed up in a gridlock or perhaps a series of roadblocks and detours on your own energetic highway that slows or stops the natural circulation of energy. We all have a highway of qi, and we all benefit from smooth-flowing qi on that highway. There are so many practices we can use to move our qi, such as tai chi, qi gong, dao yin exercises, yoga, or kung fu.

Many times when these blocks occur, they are normal reactions to life's challenges. This can lead to people feeling unwell or highly emotional because their energy isn't flowing properly through their body's energy pathways. However, the blocks may resolve themselves as people handle their circumstances and associated emotions.

There are different kinds of blocks depending on the energetic meridians that are affected. For example, if someone hurts your feelings, or you are traumatized, you may get what we call a Heart Protector block.[4] This is a fairly common reaction, and it simply means that there is a qi blockage in your Heart Protector, otherwise known as the Pericardium meridian running through your arm. When your heart gets hurt, your system has to do its natural job of trying to protect you, which creates what we call a Heart Protector block. It's usually not a serious issue, unless it continues for some time. It usually

[4] This term comes from the Five Element Chinese Medicine tradition and is not commonly used or treated in Traditional Chinese Medicine (TCM).

comes with a feeling of defensiveness and potentially some discomfort either in the arms or perhaps a feeling of congestion in the chest, which we call chest oppression, or sometimes even a feeling of panic.

Often these types of blocks (called Channel Blocks) resolve on their own, and in some cases, even physical pain can diminish or be alleviated entirely when they do, bringing more balance and a greater sense of ease. But in other cases, these blocks linger, sometimes for years. When these meridians are chronically blocked, it may be difficult to live your authentic life.

Channel Blocks are fairly commonplace. The good news is that addressing and clearing these blocks through Chinese Medicine points can be immensely beneficial to our health and happiness on every level. By restoring the natural flow of qi, many people experience significant physical and emotional improvements.

However, there can be more serious blocks in the energy system that operate on much deeper levels than simply the flow of your qi through the meridians. These profound barriers are the result of what Chinese Medicine refers to as Xie qi, which loosely translates as "evil qi," or what we prefer to call "not true qi." In essence, this implies that your authentic life energy, or your "true qi" has been subverted by some type of internal or external force.

External influences include: climatic influences such as wind or dampness, stressful energy you pick up from the world around you, which we call chaotic energy (also termed aggressive energy in Five Element Chinese Medicine), or perhaps even an entity that gets in and tries to take over.

Internal factors are found within you, such as a long-term negative emotional state or the long-term coping mechanisms that resulted from past trauma (PTSD).

These blocks can persist for long periods of time, even many years, and often require specific treatments for their removal. In Chinese Medicine there are a number of Alchemical treatments that address these kinds of *Xie* qi blocks, including the Thirteen Ghost Points treatment.

It's important to note that there's nothing intrinsically evil about *Xie* qi even though it's often translated as "evil qi," aside from the fact that it's a form of energy that's in the wrong place. It simply needs to be purged or relocated outside of the body. This can be viewed as similar to performing an exorcism, where the entity or *Gui* is guided "home" where it belongs, which many may think of as the white light or a godly realm.

Once we identify the type of block a person has, a Chinese Medicine practitioner can determine protocols to remove these blocks. The effects of clearing a block can be immediate, especially if it's some simple chaotic energy that got into your energy meridian system and caused a disturbance. A person might feel immediately better, sometimes within seconds!

The clearing of a deeper *Xie* qi block might take much longer. Often it can take three to six months for someone to rediscover their own authentic energetic self. It takes time for the person's body, mind, and spirit to shed the habits that were acquired when they were living life inauthentically. During this time, it helps to have additional support from different healing modalities to rebuild and bolster the person's true qi and true nature.

One way to think of this is that we all have our true authentic nature, which is animated by our true qi. When *Xie* qi infiltrates the system, our true qi finds it difficult to circulate through the system and therefore eventually it becomes difficult for our true nature to remain in charge of the system. Treatments like the Ghost Points attempt to reestablish the true qi so a person's true nature can "take charge of the being."[5]

---

[5] Claude Larre and Elizabeth Rochat de la Vallee, *Rooted in Spirit: The Heart of Chinese Medicine* (Barrytown, NY: Station Hill Press, 1995).

So what exactly are these deeper blocks or *Xie* qi blocks?

1. **Emotional/Trauma Hooks**: These blocks are often the result of haunting emotional or traumatic experiences from the past, often accompanied by obsessive thinking. This is why we call them "hooks," because it's as if you've been caught on a fish hook that you cannot easily wriggle free from. The Thirteen Ghost Points provide an effective Alchemical protocol for healing at this level.

2. **Heart Pains:** These blocks stem from our attempts to protect ourselves from the pain of our emotional and physical injuries in this lifetime. They are like a kind of "baggage" that accumulates in the void of the heart as we attempt to ensure that we will never have to experience certain intense life pains again. We will discuss the Heart Pains treatment protocol further in Appendix 1 of this book.

3. **Disconnected Heart Block:** These blocks often indicate that a person is unable to connect with their own heart or the hearts of the people around them. While the Thirteen Ghost Points can be an effective tool for these kinds of blocks, another powerful approach involves a different protocol, known as the *Internal Devils*, the *Internal Dragons*, or *IDs*. This specialized technique is designed to unlock a person's heart, restoring access to the spirit residing within it. We will discuss this protocol in further depth in Appendix 2 of this book.

4. **Obstructed Will Block:** This block is typically indicated when the person is unable to exert their own will and pursue their own life's aspirations. While the Thirteen Ghost Points can be an effective approach for addressing these kinds of blocks, another potent method involves another protocol, called the *External Devils*, the *External Dragons*, or EDs. These help

unshackle the person's energetic feet so that they can begin to walk their true road in life. We will discuss this protocol further in Appendix 3 of this book.

5. **Chaotic Energy Block:** These blocks present with a host of bizarre symptoms caused by chaos in the system. Over time, this chaos disrupts the qi's ability to circulate in the system, consequently limiting the free expression of the person's authenticity. We will further discuss this protocol in Appendix 4 of this book.

The Hooks That Haunt Us

The most common obstacles we may encounter are emotional or trauma-related "hooks" that literally haunt us in our lives. These emotional or traumatic sticking points can have a profound impact on our capacity to be (or not be) vulnerable and open emotionally. They often play a role in triggering our fundamental fears, misgivings, and mistrust, limiting how freely and happily we can live our lives.

After an impactful negative event happens in our lives, most of us usually want to insure that it will never, ever, ever happen again! Then, when we encounter moments that remind us even slightly of these negative past events, we tend to fear that the past will repeat itself, and we react or fail to react accordingly. This is the definition of a trigger. A trigger is something in the present making us fear a repetition of past events.

Triggers are extremely common in all of our lives. It's nearly impossible to spend much time on Earth without accumulating a few. The Thirteen Ghost Points can be incredibly effective at helping release these triggers. Given their prevalence, we advocate the use of the Thirteen Ghost Points treatments for anyone who has faced trauma or negative experiences. This approach is a significant shift from Traditional Chinese Medicine perspectives in modern times, which typically reserve the Ghost Points for addressing severe mental illness.

No Hierarchy of Trauma

In Chinese Medicine philosophy, a "ghost," a *Gui*, can be something from the past that comes back to haunt our thoughts and to even make us behave in ways we wouldn't naturally do. These triggers usually pop up intermittently or sometimes even remain activated under the surface, causing a constant state of anxiety without a lot of consciousness as to why we're feeling nervous or afraid.

The question is: how long will the effects of the trauma last and how serious are these effects? Most energy blocks, as we explained earlier, should resolve themselves relatively quickly once treated. For instance, if you are injured in a bicycle accident, you might regain the courage to ride again following your recovery, letting go of any fears that you have. Through the process of confronting your fears, you can release the block that this trauma caused and be free to enjoy riding again. Obviously, this is a best case scenario, and easier said than done for a lot of people. But for some people, the trauma gets "hooked" more deeply into them, so that in effect they have a ghost from the past still haunting their daily lives.

It's difficult to compare traumas. And there truly is no hierarchy. One person's bike accident could be as traumatic as a sexual assault to another person in terms of the way they are compromised by the experience.

This is where the Thirteen Ghost Points approach can be a really powerful modality to dissolve the emotional trauma hooks that prevent us from being free and authentically ourselves. Every person is potentially susceptible to being ensnared by these kinds of emotional or traumatic hooks. Once a thought or emotion becomes intertwined with your psyche or energy matrix, it behaves like a parasite, sapping your vital energy.

While it can be challenging to unhook emotionally and physically from traumatic events, it is not impossible and that is the focus of the rest of this book. The Thirteen Ghost points were designed to liberate us from these emotional hooks. Each of the points represents a specific vulnerability or entry point for becoming ensnared.

Emotional/trauma hooks can come from various sources:

- **PTSD:** Traumatic events can potentially create post-traumatic stress disorder (PTSD) responses. This means that when confronted with triggers reminiscent of a past trauma, a person may react as if the initial trauma is recurring, which is in essence a loss of choice, and an inability to be free and authentic in present time. For example, if a person has experienced violence, PTSD may be the result, making them feel that violence is an ongoing threat in their daily life. We see this kind of PTSD cycle among soldiers returning from war or victims of childhood abuse.

- **Negative mental patterns:** These often start with fear stemming from negative remarks or self-generated thoughts that deviate from a person's authentic self. When someone repeatedly labels you as a bad person, the negative thought can embed itself deeply within your psyche, affecting your entire sense of self. Such thoughts can lead to obsessive thinking, anxiety, depression, paranoia, compulsive behaviors, and even self-harm. While negative thoughts are a part of daily life, they usually don't persist unless we have pre-existing "hooks" from past experiences. These hooks often originate from abusive parents, grandparents, siblings, or romantic partners. Negativity can infiltrate our minds like a parasitic worm, establishing powerful mental patterns. Curses, for example, can create enduring mental patterns that are difficult to break and can last for generations.

- **Cellular patterns:** These patterns manifest as enduring, chronic physical conditions that can defy healing. Often clients with these physical issues have tried everything: pharmaceuticals, alternative medicine, psychotherapy, and any number of other modalities to attempt to heal. Any disease that's really stuck and seemingly "untreatable" is a hook. This is similar to the way a parasite lingers in the body, sometimes even after multiple treatments have been attempted. The true underlying cause of this dilemma is not actually the strength or tenacity of the parasite; rather, it resides in emotional issues that weaken your ability to heal. A compelling example is Lyme disease: many people swiftly rebound after a simple round of antibiotics, whereas others grapple with prolonged chronic Lyme disease, unable to expel the spirochetes entirely. Other prevalent and common ailments function in a similar vein, such as chronic fatigue syndrome, fibromyalgia, and migraines, as well as autoimmune diseases such as rheumatoid arthritis, ulcerative colitis, and Crohn's disease.

Releasing Emotional/Traumatic Hooks

Freeing yourself from emotional and traumatic hooks can be a challenging endeavor. Certainly it is possible to achieve without receiving a Thirteen Ghost Points treatment. However, to free yourself on your own requires substantial dedication and being constantly vigilant with your own mind.

The first step towards releasing yourself from the clutches of the emotional hooks that may be haunting you from the past involves keenly observing your own life and cultivating an awareness of all the triggers that ignite your inner "ghosts." You must identify the recurring patterns of thought and emotions that have ensnared you. For many people this is very challenging to do alone.

The next step demands unwavering attentiveness, or what we like to call "vigilance within your own mind," so that you can begin to change your default behaviors. Whenever you encounter a fear that inhibits the pursuit of your desires and even prompts you to do things you'd rather not do (like compulsive eating or drinking), it becomes imperative to shift out of that old, entrenched pattern. You must observe your emotional responses. For instance, if you consistently experience anger and frustration every time a certain trigger occurs, it becomes crucial to seek alternative ways of reacting. Instead of feeling defensive, for example, you could allow for a feeling of vulnerability and make space for some curiosity about why you are being triggered.

Experiencing the hook itself is challenging enough, but transforming old habits into new habits requires that you find a way to transform deeply ingrained patterns. Unhooking just one of these deeply entrenched hooks through a means other than Chinese Medicine's Ghost Point treatments can take years of unrelenting effort.

In light of how arduous this process can be, the Thirteen Ghost Points treatment holds immense promise in helping people overcome such entrenched patterns. When a practitioner and client work through all the Ghost Points in the protocol, the treatment goes beyond addressing one hook at a time. The Ghost Points are designed to tackle a number of hooks at the same time. These hooks are often intertwined like a jumbled, tangled ball of yarn. Even if you've been investing considerable effort into your healing journey by tugging on one of the threads, you might not be able to extricate it from the knotted mess of other strands. Anyone who's managed to unravel a complicated knot understands that most of the time you have to address the whole snarled enmeshment at once in order to free any individual string. This is the power and the wonderment of doing all of the Thirteen Ghost Points in a single, day-long treatment. It allows us to examine and untangle the whole ball of yarn, so to speak. In this way, Thirteen Ghost Points can even release the reason that you became hooked in the first place.

Putting the SELF in Self-Cultivation

Over the course of the many years we've spent teaching the Ghost Points to practitioners, we've learned that the magic of these points isn't simply in the point locations or the needling techniques. Rather, it deeply resides in our own self-cultivation. Whether you're delving into these points for individual spiritual practice or integrating them into your healing practice, we've found that the most effective means to utilize them is through a process of cultivation in which meditations, exercises, and experiences allow you to develop a close relationship with each point. Our intention is that this book will serve as a guide to an experiential journey of deeper self-cultivation. Our hope is that you will move beyond the concepts and intellectual theory to really engage these points actively and reap the rewards of the meditations and inner work it offers.

The Ghost Points come to life by bringing consciousness to habitually unconscious aspects of ourselves. There is great power in such mindful inquiry and release. Anyone willing to courageously examine their inner wounds and negativity can benefit from the teachings inherent in these points.

We often say that by age twenty, most of us carry emotional wounds and limiting "ghostly" patterns from negative experiences or trauma that imprint on us during our formative years. Some of us escape childhood with only minor hooks, while the majority of us have more extensive accumulated patterns from the past. Either way, few of us consciously process these buried hurts and conditioning, and so they persist.

This book is intended to guide you through various states of mind and to shine light into your own dark corners to help you integrate denied and disowned parts of yourself, so that you can expand into greater wholeness. The meditations in this book are designed to help you confront your unconscious ghosts, hooks, and past traumas in order to reclaim agency over your own inner world. Each reflection and exercise serves as Alchemical fire that can transform what binds you to your past so that you might fully claim and inhabit your present.

Partnering with an Alchemical practitioner can offer profound support, insightful guidance, and potentially accelerate your transformative journey—especially when you've been locked out of your own heart and need help finding the keys.

Leora Esterra, MD, one of our Master Alchemy Apprenticeship Program (MAAP) graduates explains it this way:

> *From my years now in the MAAP program, I consider self-cultivation to be a cornerstone of my practice. However, there is a magic that arises from a person receiving a Ghost Points treatment. In both observing and practicing these treatments, I have seen, over and over again, the transformation of all involved when one Heart witnesses another Heart's desire to truly know itself.*
>
> *In receiving this treatment, with a practitioner by our side, we have the opportunity to see our true selves reflected back to us in the eyes, the words, and the void of the Heart. No matter what arises, no matter what trauma or delusion comes in and takes over our minds, the loving witness by our side reminds us to return to what is true. We are here for each other, to be the other set of eyes and ears when our own might be clouded. This is the gift of being a human traveling with other humans in this mysterious world of ours, and this gift is not to be taken lightly. It is a gift that has the potential to fundamentally change the trajectory of our lives. One day we are*

receiving treatment, another day we are the practitioner.

Each time we are together, the Divine joins us in our quest so that the sum of you and me is not just the two of us. Through the magic of the Love that runs through these points, we add up to the whole of the Universe. In this paradox of an equation, an unexpected cauldron is fashioned, and between us a special kind of Alchemy arises. The Ghost Points reflect truth back to whomever walks along with them. For both sincerely seeking self-cultivators and practitioners who are self-cultivating, they guide us and reveal secrets that we find that we have always known, but somehow have forgotten.

Whether you choose to work with a practitioner or embark on this journey solo, the ultimate transformation is yours to create. This book serves as a mirror, helping you to identify and correct the distortions that have clouded your life's clarity. By doing so, you'll be able to refocus and consciously choose your path forward, free from the shadows of your past.

There is no single right (or wrong) way to transform. The pathways of transformation are as unique as the individuals traversing them. When you work with the Ghost Points with conscious intent, doing the steps in order, following their roadmap, and staying engaged with them, you will begin to free yourself from your own hooks.

One key for staying engaged and moving throughout the process is to not just passively receive these treatments, but instead, to actively participate by very consciously doing the meditations, visualizations, affirmations, and exercises that we have created specifically for each of the Ghost Points. This turns the points from being simply abstract concepts into solid tools for transformation.

The habits of life can take quite some time to unravel. Keep in mind that this is not a race but rather an adventure—a personal and sacred journey of self-cultivation from darkness to light. This book aims to demystify the ancient Thirteen Ghost Points, transforming them into practical tools for your own transformation.

Using the Ghost Points for Your Own Self-Cultivation Journey

In Chinese Medicine, we typically use points for their particular point "functions," meaning the way the point is designed to address particular symptoms or indications. For example, Spleen 1, one of the Ghost Points, when used as a primary channel acupuncture point, is good for symptoms like bloody stools and abdominal distension. The functions of the point include the ability to stop bleeding and regulate the Spleen, which in turn addresses the distension.

When we use any point as a Ghost Point, we are working in a totally different paradigm. No matter which point we choose, we are attempting to break up stuck patterns and get rid of what doesn't belong to us (ghosts and worms for example). We use each point to free ourselves from any patterns that interfere with our ability to be our most authentic selves.

Each point has a theme, so when we select a point, we are not necessarily choosing it because of its point function within a meridian, like Spleen 1's ability to stop bleeding. We select a Ghost point specifically because of the theme of the point. So Spleen 1, when used as a Ghost Point, is called Ghost Eyes. It relates to how we see the world. So treating that point releases negative patterns that influence how we see the world.

When you are in the process of self-cultivating the Ghost Points, you are taking your time with yourself, asking yourself deep questions, and then most importantly, allowing yourself the time you need to shift things... things that you may have thought you could never shift before. This requires that you give yourself permission to change even the things that might feel terrifying to look at when you first begin.

As you work through this book, give yourself some time and space not just to learn the points intellectually, but also to engage with the points inside yourself. Even the points at the end of the sequence, which are often for more serious cases, are incredibly helpful and freeing for everyone who wishes to fully clear the skeletons from their closet and embrace their newly found authenticity.

As we work through each point, we will provide a meditation to help you engage the point more deeply. We recommend that you try the meditations and adapt them however you feel will be most helpful for you. We are all different, and when we do these treatments in person, we often adapt to whatever situation the point brings up. Since we're not there in person, holding your hand and treating the points, we cannot know what that particular situation will be. You will be both the practitioner and the recipient for yourself. So we recommend that you be kind, present, and loving with yourself as you work through these points.

Witnessing Your Life

The first place to start is by taking time every day to step out of your normal mindset and watch yourself as you're living your life. We often refer to Eckhart Tolle's idea of becoming "the watcher" of your own life.[6] As the watcher, you carefully witness your life, tracking your inner and outer realities as you work through your Alchemical process. You may watch yourself let go of the self-doubt that the Ghost Convincing

---

[6] Eckhart Tolle, *The Power of Now* (Vancouver and Novato, CA, Namaste Publishing and New World Library, 1999).

point helps you release. Or you may see yourself embracing your innocence with the help of Ghost Hidden. You may see yourself discovering your true identity, beyond the trappings of the outer world, through Ghost Seal. When we work through the Ghost Points, we become watchers of the transformations we are experiencing.

Alchemical Meditation

Alchemical meditation cultivates an inward focus, sometimes called *Nei Gong* or "Inner Alchemy." This inner orientation is essential because consolidating and circulating qi in the body-mind requires practice and patience.

Whether you're new to meditation or already have an established practice, this section can help you embrace the visualization techniques that we created based on traditional Daoist approaches we have studied and learned over the years. We've designed the first meditation in this book specifically as a foundation for all the subsequent meditations, so it represents the core starting place for everyone.

If you have tried to meditate in the past but have found it difficult to sustain, many people have told us this type of visualization-based meditation is much easier for them to do. We strongly encourage you to begin with this simple relaxation meditation. Or feel free to create one of your own that similarly walks you through a relaxation visualization. There is no one way to meditate. Everyone needs to find their own way to sit in silence and begin a deeper conversation with themselves.

Alchemical meditation is a good place to start your practice, and a good place to come back to as a touchstone if you wander off your path.

Relax Your Body and Clear Your Mind Meditation—Everyone Starts Here

This relaxation technique provides the foundation for every other meditation in this book.

We recommend practicing this meditation for 15 minutes daily; first thing in the morning is optimal. Through regular practice, you will learn to quickly enter a relaxed state before moving to more advanced meditations. Once you become familiar with the steps, you may only need a few minutes to settle into a calm presence. You may also extend this up to 20 minutes in the beginning of your practice sessions.

You may listen to a similar recorded meditation we called *Relax Your Body, Clear Your Mind, and Open Your Doors* as a companion to this book at the Alchemy Learning Center website: AlchemyLearningCenter.com.

The goal of this meditation is to let go of your resistance by relaxing your body and clearing your mind, so that you may (optionally) open all the doors of possibilities in life. In order to attain the inner focus common to all Alchemical meditations, you must begin to lessen your focus on your outer experiences of the world. Once your body and mind are in a calm and clear state, it will be easier to open up to different types of meditation in the future. But this meditation is for this very moment in time.

This meditation is often done from the top down (though it can also be done from the feet up to the head, which is more energizing). We recommend that you begin with the top down approach because it has a more calming effect, starting with your head, then moving through your torso, and finally ending with your legs and feet.

Let's begin...

Sit comfortably in a chair with your feet on the floor and your hands resting on your thighs near your knees. If you wish to sit cross-legged on the floor, let your hands rest in your lap in this simple hand mudra (hand formation): Create a small bowl with the palm of one hand, and put the back of your other hand inside it, as if you're ready to accept heaven's gifts. Rain is traditionally considered a gift from heaven, so you can imagine gently falling rain pooling into your cupped hands. You can optionally touch the tips of your thumbs together.

Traditionally for males (or those who have yang-dominant energy), the left (or yang) hand rests in the right hand. For females (or those who have yin-dominant energy), the right (or yin) hand rests in the left hand.

Close your eyes and take a slow breath in, counting slowly to four, and release it slowly to a count of four.

As you breathe in again, focus on the top of your head. On your exhale, imagine that a thick liquid, like honey or maple syrup, warm and soft, is slowly moving down from the top of your head over your face and the back of your head. Feel the downward energy moving from the top of your head over your eyes.

As you breathe in again, continue to allow the energy or imagined liquid to descend down your face, making sure that any area that feels tight in your face relaxes with your exhale. Pay special attention to your eyes, your cheekbones, and your jaw. Feel all the facial muscles relax and let go.

Breathe in again and as you exhale, continue to allow a downward motion of this energy or liquid to descend down through your neck and across the tops of your shoulders and into your chest and upper back.

Breathe in again and as you exhale, visualize the energy or liquid traveling down your back and along the sides of your ribs, like a gentle waterfall, falling down all the way to your hips. As the energy reaches your hips, imagine that the downward energy is anchoring you safely into your chair or onto the floor.

From the hips, continue to allow the energy or liquid to travel down the back of your legs into your feet and into the ground. Feel your feet getting heavier as if they're connected to the ground or if you're sitting cross-legged, imagine your ankles and feet melting into the ground.

As you breathe in again, scan your body for any tension or resistance that may remain and allow that area to relax with your exhale.

Take a few minutes to clear your mind and allow this relaxation to settle into your body, mind, and spirit.

When you are finished, slowly open your eyes and see the present moment around you.

Breathe slowly. You may want to smile. You are right where you need to be at this very moment. You are now ready to begin whatever meditation you are currently working on.

The Five Elements, the Nine Palaces of The Heart, and the Magic Square

Before we go any deeper into explaining the Alchemy journey, we first want to be sure that you're somewhat familiar with three major Chinese philosophical concepts we'll be referencing throughout the book. For us, these concepts are key to your Alchemical journey and may offer deeper insights into your quest for more understanding of the Thirteen Ghost Points.

We have laid out a (very) brief overview of these important concepts in this section. Please feel free to refer to this section as you're reading through the book, as we will mention these ideas numerous times. If you would like more information about these concepts, please visit the Alchemy Learning Center at AlchemyLearningCenter.com and view the Free Access section.

- **The Five Elements:** This is the way we describe the five essential types of energetic movement throughout the universe. The energy of every being on the planet is found in the Five Elements, which are Wood, Fire,

Earth, Metal, and Water. This is the cornerstone of much of our Alchemical philosophy, and many ancient Daoist texts reference these five energies, dating back to the earliest Confucian writings.

- **The Nine Palaces of the Heart a.k.a. The Nine Heart Pains:** These are the nine essential parts of our lives that must be attended to so that we can live in balance and attain peace. The Nine Palaces (listed below) consist of nine lessons for every human being of how to live life, a simple yet profound roadmap. Attention to each of the Nine Palaces is the basis for how we can obtain a feeling of satisfaction or completion in life so that we can die with, what the Daoists call, "no unfinished business," which basically means with no regrets. We discuss the Nine Heart Pains Treatment in Appendix 1 of this book.

- **The Magic Square:** According to legend, the Nine Palaces were created by Yu the Great, who found a mystical numerical pattern called the Magic Square on the back of a turtle who showed up after a great flood.

The Five Elements

The Five Elements are based on the concepts of yin and yang. Yang Energy is energy that travels upward and outward. Yin Energy is energy that travels downward and condenses inward. Because yang and yin are in constant motion and flux, the Five Elements define five different ways that yang and yin energies play out in the world. Here is a short intro into each Element.

- **Wood:** When yang energy rises out of yin, it has an upward strong energy that can break through barriers. However, like a sprout in the Spring, it is ultimately a little fragile. Wood energy is out front—a leader with strong opinions, who likes to spearhead new projects. Wood energy moves with spurts of forward motion, then retreats and regroups before moving forward again.

- **Fire:** When the yang energy reaches its pinnacle, it begins to branch out and starts to tip downward into Yin, like a flower opening and blooming in mid-Summer. Social, energized, optimistic, needing to be admired and loved, focused on beauty and harmony, the Fire Element type wants to be the lover in the world. Fire energy moves upward and then downward in an unpredictable manner, always in the process of either lifting or falling.

- **Earth:** When the yin and yang energy are balanced, we have the Earth element. Social, community-oriented, care-taking, and hospitable, Earth Element individuals are at the center of everything, and they function as the glue that holds us all together. Earth energy is flowing circularly in its movement, either moving inward to the center or moving outward to the periphery.

- **Metal:** When yin Energy begins descending out of yang Energy, it has a withdrawn aspect but is still a force to be reckoned with. Observant, conscientious, exacting, conserving, and deserving of respect, the Metal Element individual wants to connect in whole-hearted sincerity (a cosmic connection) or not at all. Metal energy is a falling downward movement that appears effortless.

- **Water:** When yin energy condenses to its furthest downward point, it gathers power to shoot up into yang again. Water alternates between quiet and resting for long periods, followed by periods of intensity. Water Element types want to matter to others and ultimately, to themselves as well. Water energy is consistently changeable and flows in a relentless forward movement that can be gentle or powerful, slow or fast, temporarily still, or constantly rapid.

As we begin to introduce you to each of the Thirteen Ghost Points, you'll see that depending on your Elemental nature, you will have a resonance or even a vulnerability based on different Ghost Points.

The Nine Palaces of the Heart

The Nine Palaces are the nine areas of a human's life that must be attended to for a sense of fulfillment and completion in life. Sometimes we call this your curriculum for a given lifetime. The Palaces are sometimes referred to as the Nine Heart Pains, because when we are unable to achieve fulfillment in any one or more of them, it can cause much heart pain. Here's a short description of each palace.

- **Career/Knowledge**: The knowledge you gather is put together into skills that then become your career, which is the way you offer yourself to the world. It's a Water Element palace.

- **Love/Relationship**: We begin life with relationships we are given through our birth circumstances. However, as we become independent, we have choices about who we choose for our relationships. Love and unconditional love experiences belong here. It's a Fire Element palace.

- **Health/Wellness**: The most basic and fundamental of all the palaces, our Health is paramount to our survival.

We may choose to protect our health or perhaps endanger it or simply ignore it. This palace is an important starting point for everyone. The strength of our health palace is key to our ability to acquire good experiences in all other palaces. It's a Wood Element palace.

- **Wealth/Abundance**: Having a sense of abundance, regardless of how much money or material objects you have accumulated, is the core issue here. Being able to allow abundance to flow to you is the focus of this palace. It can be challenging to unravel the ultimate truth of our Wealth Palace due to the prevalence of materialistic values in our modern society. It's a Wood Element palace.

- **Home/Connection to Divine**: Having a sense of belonging and peace in your life is what the Home Palace is all about. We like to call it, "Home with a capital H." Even though this is the fifth Palace, it's considered the most advanced as it holds the center position of the Magic Square below, which means that before your life's journey transitions towards completion, you must attend to your spiritual Home for a sense of fulfillment in life. It's an Earth Element palace.

- **Travel/Global/Adventure**: A sense of adventure and a knowing that people all around the world are fundamentally the same—that's the spirit of the Travel Palace. The global perspective is a way of seeing that we are all sharing the same experience, but each person comes to it from a unique individual perspective. The commonality of human experience is key here. It's a Metal Element palace.

- **Children/Creativity/Legacy**: This palace concerns our ability to create new life as humans, as well as all the ways we may relate to our creations of every kind. How will your creations be viewed by others in future generations? What will your legacy be? Think of this palace as the cosmic ripple you've made in the universal pool of time and space. There's a sense here of destiny and that either something is meant to be, or it's not. It's a Metal Element palace.

- **Wisdom/Inner Knowing**: We gather knowledge through studies and experiences, but we don't achieve wisdom until it coalesces into a deeper knowing. This palace differs from the Career/Knowledge Palace in the sense that Wisdom flows from living and having experiences, not necessarily from book learning or the acquisition of skills. It's a Water Element palace.

- **Prosperity/Charity**: From our sense of abundance, a deep desire to give back to the world is born—a sense of generosity and a desire to share for the betterment of future generations. This palace can be a challenge for many people, yet it is foundational for human existence. Think of acquiring wealth or resources like time, money, fuel, or land, and freely giving this bounty to those who may be in need, without any strings attached. Can you detach freely and willingly from what you have in order for someone who has less than you to receive? It's a Fire Element palace.

The Magic of the Magic Square

The ancient Chinese legend of the Magic Square tells of a great flood tamed by the heroic Yu the Great. He ingeniously channeled floodwaters into the earth through holes that he drilled with his staff. After this feat, a mystical tortoise

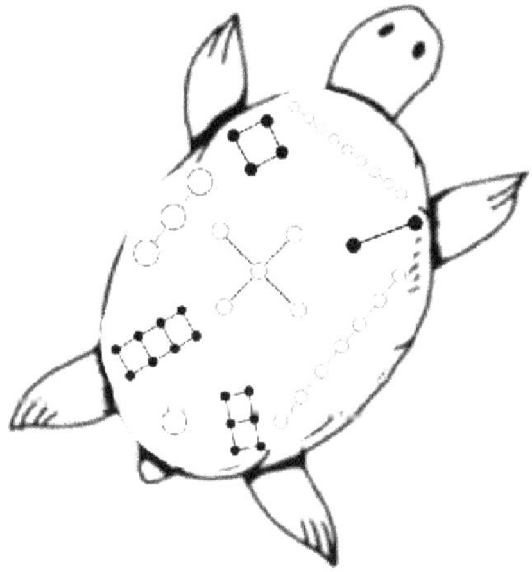

emerged from the river Lo with a strange pattern on its shell.

The pattern, known as the *Lo Shu* or "magic square," was made up of strange and curious markings that turned out to be more than just an interesting design. Yu observed a grid that contained rows and columns of linked dots – where all the rows and columns within the grid added up to the same sum: the number fifteen – like magic!

The numerology of the Magic Square became linked to the Daoist concept of the Nine Palaces, with each square being associated with one of the nine life themes or lessons.

One way you can think of the Magic Square is that it's like a game board, where the objective of the game is to get to the center square—the Home Palace. But before you can journey Home, you first have to patiently complete your assigned tasks at each of the outer squares. In Daoist theory, the Nine Palaces magic square is like a mandala for self-realization. Its magical numbering system points to a path of perseverance (in the same way that Yu persisted to conquer the great flood for years) that will lead to enlightenment or the ability to find your spiritual Home at the center.

MAGIC SQUARE

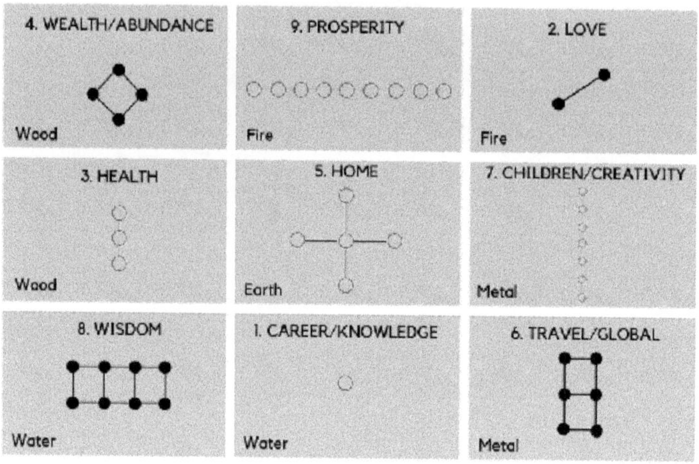

The path through the Nine Palaces in your life begins at the bottom center with the first palace, the Career/Knowledge Palace, and proceeds in numerical order to the Love Palace, the Health and Wealth Palaces, (skipping the fifth Palace), and continues through the rest of the next eight areas of life. Once you've finished your eighth palace, you can gain access to the final square in the center, which was given the number five, which is exactly halfway between the number one and the number nine. Therefore, the Home Palace, number five—the one that's in the center of all the others—is actually the last palace in your Nine Palace curriculum.

Five Elements and Nine Palaces for Self-Cultivation

As we said earlier, we wanted you to begin to understand a few of the basic principles of Alchemy and Chinese Medicine philosophy before we dive into the Ghost Points. Whether you're a practitioner or a life-long learner interested in deepending your Wisdom Palace, we can't think of a better place to start your journey than understanding your Five Elements and Nine Palaces.

In this book, we invite you to peek behind your own Home Palace door. Who are you? What is your authentic nature? Understanding this in yourself is the perfect place to start before diving deep into the mysteries of the Thirteen Ghost Points. If you wish, you can visit the Alchemy Learning Center at AlchemyLearningCenter.com and listen to the free *Who Am I* Alchemical Meditation.

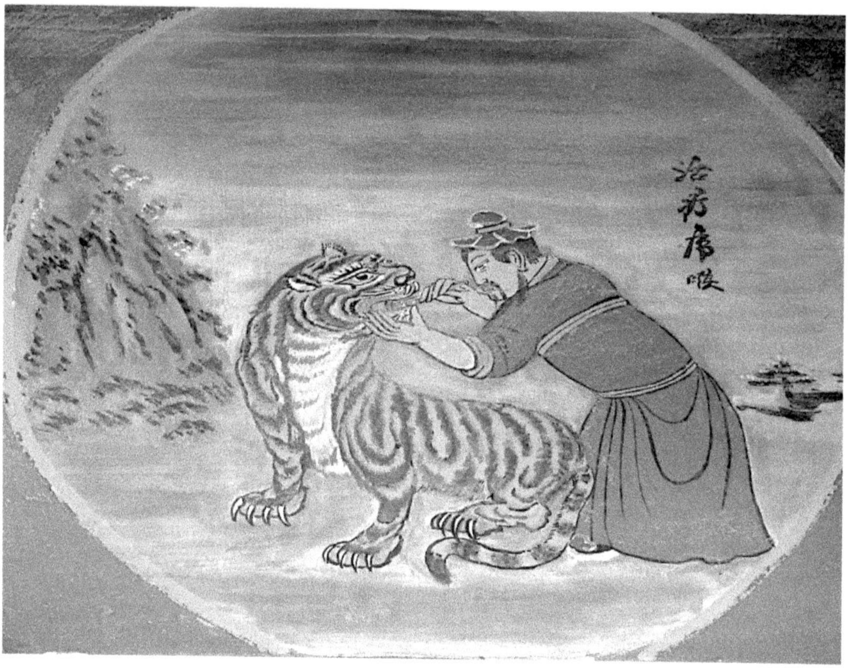

Sun SiMiao saving a tiger, Huanglong Temple, LuoFu Shan, Guangdong, China

PART TWO:
For Practitioners

This section introduces you to the philosophy behind becoming an Alchemical Practitioner or what we like to call an Alchemical Facilitator. It also invites you to examine the kind of practitioner you are and want to be.

You must first have a deep understanding of your own life before pretending to know life in another, especially the disturbances in the development of life in another.

—*Claude Larre and Elizabeth Rochat de Vallée*

Chapter Three: Becoming an Alchemical Facilitator

For many practitioners, Alchemical Chinese Medicine is a brand new mindset, even if it is thousands of years old. It breaks the old paradigm of the role of the medical professional, which has dictated that "the doctor knows best," and has insisted that the patient follow the doctor's instructions, even to the point of ignoring their own instincts.

Practicing Alchemy as a practitioner is not about helping at all. In fact, in our Apprenticeship program we make everyone practice repeating the phrase: "I cannot help you" to themselves while working with clients. They repeat this over and over in their minds until they can begin to trust that their role is simply to be a facilitator in the healing session. Rather than "helping," the practitioner learns to simply trust the patient's destiny path and be the facilitator of change. The "illness" has appeared in order to provoke change, and the practitioner is now simply present to walk alongside the patient and encourage them to do what is necessary to move through the Nine Palaces curriculum, or the lessons of their lifetime.

Becoming an Alchemical Facilitator requires more than just a grasp of point location, treatment protocols, and theories regarding the progression of illnesses. While becoming a skilled technician and mastering these technical aspects is very valuable, it can also be limiting if we, as practitioners, believe that the treatment's effectiveness hinges solely on these kinds of technical elements.

In contrast, the practice of Alchemy requires a degree of spiritual self-cultivation on the part of the practitioner. This entails engaging in activities that enhance self-awareness, such as daily meditation and journaling. It also can involve many other consistent practices to nurture the body and mind, such as energy-moving exercises like tai chi, qi gong, or yoga, maintaining a healthy diet, fostering a deep connection to nature and the seasons, ensuring quality sleep, and cultivating self-love.

The Alchemy points we work with are the very same points commonly used in everyday acupuncture practices. So while it's important to know the Alchemy treatment point locations, treatment protocols and theories, it is paramount to understand that all healing has some aspect of the miraculous in it.

How else can points that are commonly used for symptoms and conditions in acupuncture become transformational Alchemy points?

The key ingredient is the practitioner!

What imbues the acupuncture points with their mystical quality is the practitioner's commitment to self-cultivation and nurturing a deep connection with both themself and the points. This dedication transforms ordinary meridian points into potent "ghost points." It is through the practitioner's journey of self-exploration that this transformation occurs.

To become an Alchemy practitioner, you must first transform and align with your true self. In this process, you must clear your own baggage, before you will be able to facilitate clearing someone else's.

> *"You must first have a deep understanding of your own life before pretending to know life in another, especially the disturbances in the development of life in another."*[7]

One crucial aspect of this journey involves embracing the state of pure presence, fully immersing yourself in the present moment without any agendas or expectations, including any assumption that a person must heal and recover.

What if the greatest growth will arise from the client's experience of being unwell? Why should we promote our agenda to make them better? Which journey—illness or wellness—will better guide them toward their true, authentic self? On many occasions, when a person has worked through their past trauma with the Ghost Points, they often surprise themselves by saying they wouldn't trade anything for their negative experiences of the past because, in the end, it's what made them who they are today.

Attaining such a profound level of presence as a practitioner can be quite a challenge. For example, can you sustain prolonged eye contact with someone that you are not intimate with? With a casual friend? With a stranger you just met? Initially, it might feel uncomfortable, but it's a crucial part of cultivating this deeper level of awareness. It entails not just listening to the words someone is saying but also at the same time sensing what the spirit wishes to convey, hidden within the essence that lies behind the words, or even within the tranquil moments when no words are being exchanged.

How connected can you be to another person's spirit and to the world around you simultaneously? It's about catching every nuance, and even noticing when the surrounding sounds, light, and movement of air are influencing the present moment.

---

[7] Claude Larre and Elizabeth Rochat de la Vallée, "The Practitioner-Patient Relationship: Wisdom from the Chinese Classics" *Journal of Traditional Acupuncture* (Winter 1990-91): 15.

For the Alchemical Facilitator, this requires attaining a state of zero ego, zero expectations, and zero thoughts and ideas about what you may think is good for the client. You are on the deeply transformational ride right along with them. This is a radical way to look at treating someone in a modern day healing practice.

This approach may not always come naturally to the facilitator at first, and that's perfectly fine. It's a skill that takes practice, like learning to dance to a new genre of music or learning a new language. We recommend starting as an observer and watching several treatments in person, focusing on one aspect of the treatment at a time. For example, you can observe how the facilitator navigates through the treatment at first, then you can focus on the patient's experience in a subsequent treatment, and then, in the next session, absorb the way that energy fills the whole treatment room and the interplay of light and the movement of air plus ambient sounds... all important aspects to be aware of in any treatment. Gradually, you can refine your skills and become a magician of presence—being present and open in a moment of time and space.

Becoming an Alchemical Facilitator: Is the Path Already in Front of You?

Alchemical healing goes beyond merely "helping" others—it's about your own personal evolution. You will change, transform, and even transmute. By walking alongside your clients, you'll fast-track your own personal growth through self-cultivation, self-understanding, and recognizing your own ghosts. In this journey, you'll also facilitate others in learning to do the same.

The first step in becoming an Alchemical Facilitator is to let go of the concept of being a "healer." This work is more like being a supporter who can recognize that each one of your clients is already inherently perfect. In fact, we are each **born perfect**. As human beings, we all possess unique qualities that set us apart from others, even if we are striving to conform. It's the Alchemical Facilitator's job to see the entire person as a divine being. Even as they tell the story of their imperfect moments, you maintain an awareness of their inherent perfection.

When you take on or assume the role of facilitator, you begin to understand that life itself can sometimes throw people off their course. This is where the magic of Alchemy comes into play. Through a profound sense of presence, we can subtly nudge our clients on their journey to their innate perfection, to their authentic selves, all without any specific agenda or a compulsion to heal them, which in the end only they can do for themselves. With the underlying agenda of wanting to fix things, which is so much a part of modern medicine, we can become too fixated on the healing, taking us out of being fully present in the moment. It's hard to deviate from this healer paradigm, especially when you show up for a day-long Ghost Point treatment, and you have to simply release any attachment to the client getting better. That's a challenge.

Why would you want to do this? Because deep emotional healing requires being present, without expectations. We're after "the real deal," not just surface-level improvements. We're stripping away the agendas. This is the secret ingredient to being an Alchemical Facilitator and the fundamental foundation of your Alchemical journey. You must give up being a "helper" and instead simply be one hundred percent you, with full eye contact, walking the path side-by-side with another human being.

The Alchemical approach is similar to working with the Eight Extraordinary Vessels, one of the Five Channel systems of Chinese Medicine. Working with the Eight Extraordinary Vessels also can create radical change over a period of three to twelve months or so. The Eight Extraordinary Vessels approach impacts the DNA level, what we call the *Jing*/Essences in Chinese Medicine, and heals pre-birth (ancestral or past-life) influences on the physical body.

The Alchemical approach works with the magic of a person's *Shen*/Spirit, rather than focusing on the *Jing*/Essences. The *Shen*/Spirit is the guiding force for your lifetime. It's the thing that mixes with the *Jing*/Essences and "takes charge of the being." It actually sets the path of your destiny, what we call your *ShenMing*, your spirit's destiny.

Working directly with the *Shen* is where the magic of transmutation can occur. If something, someone, or some past traumatic event is holding you back or blocking your way, you can go to the root of that issue, and shift it all at once, creating immediate change. Sometimes though, while the change is immediate, it takes time for the rest of the being to catch up in order for a person to fully integrate the radical change and to release the old inauthentic habits. Undergoing this kind of change can take some getting used to, so we must allow for a period of adjustment. Depending on the person, this can take one second (literally!), a month, or most typically, three to six months or more.

If you are a Chinese Medicine practitioner or an energy healer, it's important to understand that this represents a whole new approach to Chinese Medicine, distinct from the typical teachings in the Western world or even many modern Chinese schools. As a guiding light for your clients, Alchemical Chinese Medicine can have a profound transformative impact while also catalyzing your own transformation. It is a shared journey—practitioner and client walking side by side—yet each must travel their own unique path.

Instrument of the Divine

Becoming a Ghost Points practitioner demands a dedicated effort to cultivate yourself as an instrument of the

Divine, guiding both clients and ghosts from where they are stuck to where they need to be.

The cultivation takes time. You are developing your own uprightness and self-esteem. You are encouraging your own light to shine fully and brightly so that it can be a beacon of light for your clients. To do this, you must learn to let go of your own fears because fear is yin energy, and yin energy attracts ghosts. What fears do you have? This is a question that needs to be answered. If one answer to that question is the fear of death, then it will be essential to overcome that and to recognize that death is simply a transition to another state of being.

Your *Shen*/Spirit has to be strong enough to ensure that this kind of treatment is invigorating, not draining for you. How strong is your *Shen*?

Having a kind, ethical heart is more important than having all the book learning in the world... Using the power of consciousness, your body becomes the crucible in which the positive forces of heaven are called down to cleanse the unrefined energy of the earth. This is cosmic alchemy on the grandest scale.

—Dr. Baolin Wu[8]

[8] Dr. Baolin Wu and Jessica Eckstein, *Lighting the Eye of the Dragon.* (New York: St. Martin's Press, 2000), 197-198.

Chapter Four: What Type of Practitioner Are YOU?

We all wear many hats in our lives. Wife, husband, mother, father, sister, brother... We are different in each of these roles. For this moment in time, you can ask yourself a few questions and let the answers give you an idea of what type of practitioner you are. Who are you today? Who might you be tomorrow? And what does that even mean?

The Technician/Hero

Are you a Technician/Hero? The technician delights in the precision of point locations, their functions, their meridians, the patterns of disease, as well as the technical aspects of diagnosing and treating patients. Often adopting a more heroic approach to healing, the technician uses their skills to "fix" what appears to be broken. This is where many healers begin their journey, accumulating knowledge and skills. Most schools emphasize these essential skills and foster the desire to heal (often from the heroic perspective), as both are helpful at the outset of any healer's path.

The hero wants to help the client. We all feel great when a treatment "works" and the person feels better. It makes our lives feel meaningful to think that we can help others. And this feeling can motivate us to continue along the path of becoming a healer.

Many practitioners who connect or relate to this style of healing often love the theory side of learning. They may spend their entire career enjoying the study of the classics and accumulating more knowledge about different techniques and theories. As they amass a library of knowledge, they also hone their skills and become incredibly proficient at healing.

Is this where your heart lies? If so, that's wonderful, and we believe in embracing this aspect of yourself wholeheartedly.

The Teacher/Saint

The Teacher on the other hand, may not be so concerned about all the nitty-gritty details. They're looking for that "ah-ha" moment where we can help others to learn how to do things for themselves. This is more of a saintly role.

The Saint tries to help clients to accept themselves and the world around them, fostering a sense of ease in their lives, regardless of circumstances. The Saint doesn't believe in heroic feats but rather in the importance of learning to better endure life's hardships by understanding ourselves better. They believe this self-awareness is key to becoming better human beings overall.

A clarifying distinction between the technician/hero and the teacher/saint can be framed by this question: Would you prefer to provide a treatment that alleviates someone's symptoms, or teach them a method to address these symptoms themselves, now and in the future? A technician/hero might prioritize the immediate relief of symptoms, while the teacher/saint might focus on imparting methods and lessons for self-care. Additionally, the teacher/saint may also guide individuals on how to better manage aspects of their condition that may not be easily changed.

The Shaman/Alchemist

The Shaman occupies a unique space between the technician and teacher approaches. The Shaman approach isn't solely about precision and skill, nor just about teaching and patience. Instead, the Shaman focuses on being fully present, placing them at the intersection between these two other approaches—where actual magic can occur. This is the path of the Alchemist, where inspired action meets the art of letting go, creating an extraordinary blend. A Shaman can effortlessly transition between these two roles—Technician/Hero and the Teacher/Saint—with fluidity.

Many practitioners embody aspects of all these roles. The key question is, "Which role do I truly prefer?" The role you love is the one you should embrace. While the Alchemical practitioner may not be your current focus, you may find yourself stepping into this role or transitioning through all three roles at different times. Even with the ability to shift between these roles, it's crucial to determine your preferred role to better understand your approach to health and healing.

Psychic Powers

In addition to your preferred practitioner role, it can also be important to understand your innate psychic powers. These may include clairvoyance, clairaudience, clairsentience, and claircognizance. As humans, we all have psychic powers, but some of us are more tuned into one form or the other. Some of us choose to cultivate and utilize these skills, while others may be completely unaware of them or simply opt not to use them. It is all a choice based on your perspective. Let's look at the four most recognized ways to receive energetic or other-dimensional information.

Clairvoyance: Visual

Are you clairvoyant? If so, then you're likely visual and able to see colors, shapes, and even entire stories play out like movies in your mind. This is useful as an Alchemical practitioner because the visual information you're receiving may give clues as to what needs to happen in a treatment, or may help you figure out the best timing, such as when to move on to the next point.

It's especially important for clairvoyant practitioners to understand that the visual information they receive can be incredibly specific, but what you receive is not necessarily something the client needs to know about. This is a level of communication happening between you and the Divine or even a ghost entity, and it may be quite disturbing and unhelpful to share this information with your clients. Developing discernment about what information is actually meant for your client is an important skill for all clairvoyants.

Clairaudience: Auditory

If you're clairaudient, you're more inclined to perceive psychic information through auditory means—ancestral whispers, Divine messages, or even understanding the significance of a song playing at the moment. This is a skill that requires tremendous multi-tracking in the treatment room. There are instances where you may be receiving something while simultaneously listening to something very important that the patient is saying. If you're clairaudient, it's important to be able to listen attentively to more than one stream of consciousness at a time.

It's also important, as with clairvoyance, to understand that your patient need not always be privy to everything you hear, and in fact, telling them may cause more harm than good. It's wiser to proceed with caution and refrain from sharing what you've heard until you develop the discernment of what is appropriate to share with a particular client.

Clairsentience: Touch

Clairsentience involves the ability to sense energy, physical sensations, and the subtle meaning of touch. For instance, while working with a client, you may perceive a sudden qi blockage in the body when they clam up about a specific upsetting topic. This may be a cue for you to ask questions to help them start talking again, which in turn can help the energy flow again.

Or you may use your clairsentience to feel when a point is truly done, not by noticing any external factors, but by sensing the energy under your fingers, beneath the surface anatomy of the patient.

While clairsentience is not often well known, it can sometimes be useful to share what you're noticing with a patient to affirm what the patient is feeling. When the patient feels something similar to what you're able to describe, it can validate the effectiveness of the treatment in real time. Be discerning with this so that you maintain rapport with each individual client.

Claircognizance: Psychic or Intuitive

Finally, claircognizance is a bit different. It doesn't involve the senses at all. It's just a psychic knowing. This may seem more rare, but only because it's difficult to acknowledge when you're experiencing your own personal cognizance versus a psychic download. Those who experience claircognizance can often feel the difference quite clearly between their own mind's knowledge and their actual psychic insights.

You may be someone who receives guidance or realizations from some other source, and you may not even know where it's coming from. But these realizations make up the foundation of your healer's intuition and need to be cultivated, just like any of the other psychic powers. If you suspect you have this ability, it can be very hard to understand at first, and you have to be patient with yourself as you learn how to best use it and manage it in treatments.

Knowing Yourself

Knowing your strengths and weaknesses in each of these areas can be important as you grow, develop, and cultivate yourself for your Alchemical work. It's a part of becoming a practitioner that many people do not often think about, yet, we believe it is essential in the early stages of understanding yourself as a healer. So going forward, we invite you to take some time to notice, explore, observe, see, hear, and feel.

Ethically Speaking

The Alchemical Practitioner also needs to know how to be a facilitator. We need to create and develop a deep rapport and professional intimacy with every one of our clients. This requires a tremendous amount of personal responsibility and self-cultivation on the part of the practitioner.

When working as an Alchemical Practitioner, your clients will be placing their complete trust in you as they share their deepest, most intimate stories and emotions. In return, they will expect that you will not abuse their trust. The information they share bestows a certain amount of power that you will have in their lives. Because of this, you'll need to practice high levels of confidentiality and professionalism with all your clients.

You may feel a great affinity with your clients after you share such intimate sessions together and then subsequently you may want to become their friend or trade your treatments for some kind of service they offer. From our personal experience, we believe that becoming the friend or employer of your clients in a sense robs them of their practitioner. Even asking them to help you with something in your life, like housesitting or working at your front desk, can cross boundaries.

When you cross that boundary into the friendship zone, you typically feel free to share your own intimate stories, which means that you will no longer hold the mystery for them. We don't believe in "good or bad" or say that you can never befriend a client under any circumstances, but it's important to be aware of the consequences of such an action, which is that you essentially stop being their practitioner by becoming their friend.

It's tempting to hire a lovely person to help you or to meet them for tea outside the treatment room. But we've learned through experience that the person has to change their relationship to you, and that then affects how they will receive future treatments from you.

In addition, it's tempting to be excited about Alchemy and to want all your friends to experience it as well. This is a bit more of a gray area. It can work well to do Alchemy with certain friends, and with others it can be dicey. It's helpful to feel into what's best for each individual and to not let your enthusiasm about Alchemy cloud your best judgment.

If you are a person who is very social, or if you are searching for a life partner or a bigger circle of friends, you will need to find ways to separate your personal life from your Alchemical healing work. This is challenging for many new practitioners, but with practice, determination, and a strong ethical integrity, it is achievable.

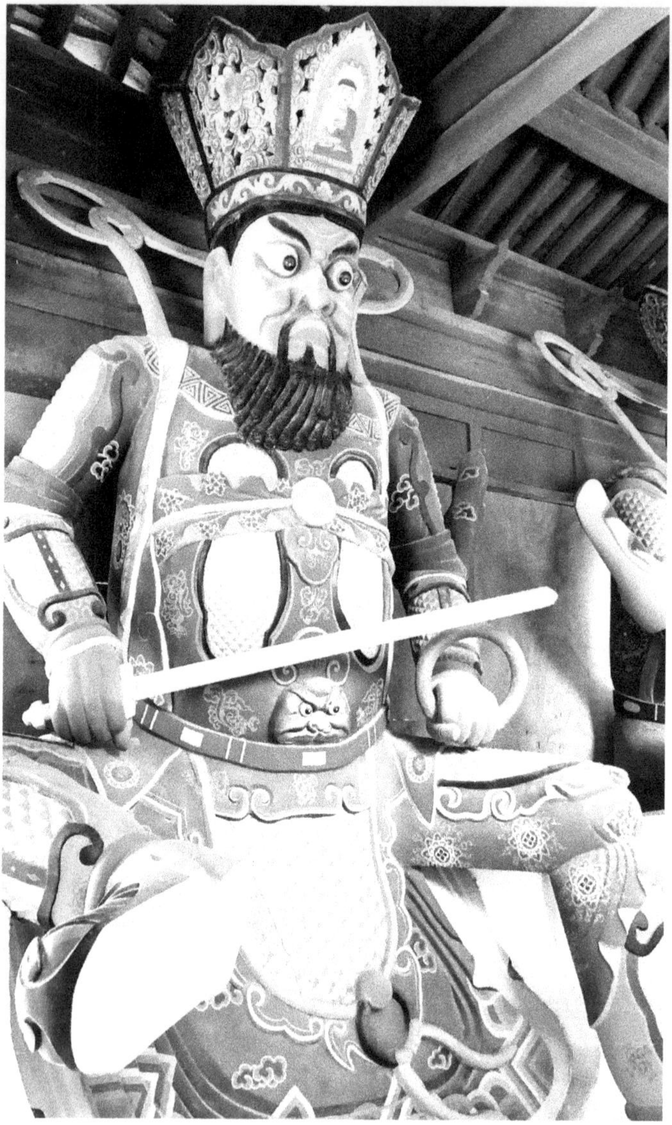

The South King, one of the Four Heavenly Kings, Leiyin Temple, Dunhuang, China

PART THREE: THE THIRTEEN GHOST POINT TREATMENT

In this section we will cover assessment techniques, treatment methods, and go over each of the Ghost Points in depth. Whether you're a practitioner or self-cultivator, we recommend that you take your time and go through the points slowly, working on yourself before you attempt to treat others as a practitioner.

Sun SiMiao's Ode of the Thirteen Ghost Points provides a list of the points with minimal instructions on their usage. The text has been interpreted in various ways by different translators and by different Chinese practitioners. The Ode reveals very few actual techniques to use. In this book, we've compiled our learning from decades of our personal research and clinically applied experience as well as our many years of studying with our teachers.

As to the reading of pulses and other techniques of diagnosis... when I heard of any man who excelled me in any of these, no distance would keep me from him. I would learn what he had to teach and then apply it.

— Sun SiMiao[9]

[9] Sun SiMiao, *Essential Formulas of Alchemical Classics*, Trans. by Nathan Sivin (1968), quoted in *Taoist Meditation and Longevity Techniques*, Ed. by Livia Kohn (Ann Arbor, MI: Center for Chinese Studies, The University of Michigan: 1989), 279.

Chapter Six: Assessment

While classical acupuncture techniques, such as pulse and tongue diagnosis, are somewhat useful for determining whether to do a Ghost Points treatment, we believe that most people who have been alive on this planet for 20 years or more would benefit from a Thirteen Ghost Points treatment.

From this perspective, we generally tend to approach our assessments more from signs and symptoms than from traditional diagnostics like taking pulses or looking at the tongue. Our focus would tend to be more looking for stuck cellular or emotional patterns, obsessions, possessions, or the sense or presence of curses.

Xie Qi – Not True Qi

In Chinese Medicine, practitioners mostly use pulse diagnosis to evaluate a person's qi/energy. However, there are a number of ways to evaluate a person's qi as it relates to assessing whether or not to do a Ghost Points treatment.

The goal of the assessment is to determine whether the person has any *Xie* qi. As we have already explained, *Xie* qi is a difficult word to describe. We like to call it "Not True" qi, meaning that the qi of the person is not exhibiting the natural movement of the person's spirit and essences. Or to put it more simply, the person's qi is not authentic. *Xie* qi is sometimes translated as evil or perverse qi, which sounds worse than it often is. We use this term to describe how a "ghost" (which can be an emotional pattern) is taking over the qi of another being or "perverting" it.

Xie qi can "get into" a person for two main reasons:

- The interior of the body/mind/spirit is vulnerable
- The exterior of the body isn't being effectively safeguarded. Exterior vulnerability can be caused by a weakened immune system or what Chinese Medicine calls weak *Wei* qi or Defensive qi.

Every now and then, even when a person has a strong exterior, life circumstances can momentarily lower their defenses, creating an opening for a "ghost" to slip into the interior. In these cases, the body's defenses may engage in a battle, the loss of which results in illness. On the other hand, people with weakened internal or external defenses may not exhibit signs of sickness when a "ghost" gets in, but still might experience strange feelings or behaviors

There are three different types of *Xie* qi blocks:

- **A Systemic Heart Block:** this manifests as the person no longer being accessible to themself or others. When this happens, we say that you've been locked out of your own heart and need help finding the keys. In this case, working with a practitioner is extremely helpful to release this block. We use the IDs treatment in this case (see *Appendix* 2).
- **A Will Block:** the person is unable to do what they want to do and so they are unable to follow their destiny. When this happens, we say your Will is blocked, and similar to a Systemic Heart block, it's extremely helpful to work with a practitioner to release this block. We use the Eds treatment in this case (see *Appendix* 3).
- **Chaotic Energy:** when chaotic energy infiltrates the body's *Wei* qi system and the proper 24 hour circulation of the *Wei* qi is disrupted. (We do not

discuss the complete treatment of this kind of *Xie* qi in this book. But see *Appendix* 4 for general information about Chaotic Energy treatments.)

In addition, there are a number of different types of internal *Xie* qi that may result in conditions such as anxiety, depression, obsessive/compulsive thinking and behavior, negative thinking (which we sometimes call "worms in the mind"), and post-traumatic stress disorder (PTSD).

Signs and Symptoms

Here are some common emotional and/or spiritual reasons to consider doing a Ghost Points treatment:

- Feeling overwhelmed by life's challenges
- Sensing a lack of freedom and autonomy in one's life
- Enduring a toxic environment in the past or present
- Navigating through a period of profound negativity in the past or present
- Being haunted by a negative thought that was implanted in the psyche
- Wrestling with haunting memories of past traumas
- Battling persistent feelings of guilt or shame stemming from past experiences

In addition, we often recommend a Ghost Points treatment for chronic health conditions, such as:

- Illness that is unresponsive to conventional treatment, especially treatments that generally work for other clients
- Autoimmune diseases
- Parasitic diseases that have become chronic conditions, such as chronic Lyme disease
- Mental illness of any type, including anxiety and

depression or "phlegm misting the heart"

The range of severity of any of these symptoms can stem from very mild, where the person has slightly deviated from their true essence/path due to mild illness or past events and thoughts, to quite severe, where the person is inaccessible to themself or the world or unable to do anything, even barely able to get out of bed.

Evaluation

There are a number of methods for assessing people on a physical level.

Pulses

A simplistic measure of the pulse is that a person's True qi overall, across all pulses, feels muffled or slippery, as if all the pulses have honey poured over them. The closest thing to this quality of pulses is when someone is pregnant; since you are feeling two beings in a single pulse, it has a similar quality.

Other qualities that might be present include:

- A beady pulse
- A knotted or irregular pulse that skips a beat felt, located on the moderate level with a nodular feeling
- A relatively slow pulse on the deep level or very rapid on the superficial level or both

Touch

A simple assessment method is to place your hand on the person to assess their energy internally.

Place your hand on the person's front side (belly or chest) and feel whether their energy is accessible to you from the front. When the person has a Heart/Yi block, it feels like cardboard, almost inert.

When you place your hand on the person's back to feel whether their energy is accessible from the back, a Will/*Zhi* block will feel like you cannot access their energy from the back; as on the front, it feels like cardboard or inert.

Complexion

Often the person's complexion may look odd or off-colored. They might look ashen or gray. There may be an odd aura around them. In Chinese Medicine, practitioners often assess the color of a person's complexion to determine their energetic type. If the person's color doesn't match their energetic type, there may be *Xie* qi present. Also note that this can cause a misdiagnosis of the person's Elemental type also known as their constitutional factor or CF.

Voice

It is not uncommon for a person's voice to sound different when *Xie* qi is present, especially if there is an actual *Gui* possession. This often becomes most apparent in a voice that sounds younger or older than the person's actual age, especially when the pitch of the voice is higher or lower than it should be.

In Chinese Medicine, practitioners often assess the sound of a person's voice to determine their energetic type. If the person's voice doesn't match their energetic type, there may be *Xie* qi present. As stated above, this can also cause a misdiagnosis of the person's Elemental type.

Eyes

The eyes are literally the windows to the spirit in Chinese Medicine and should naturally exhibit the spirit's light shining out of them. When a person has *Xie* qi, their eyes change. They may look vacant, like the person isn't home. They may simply seem odd to you, as if the person's eyes are deviated but they aren't. You may see flashes of something that comes and goes behind the eyes. You may see a fuzzy look in the eyes, almost as if the eyes are vibrating slightly. Anything that looks strange or abnormal may be *Xie* qi. We believe that everyone has the ability to see the difference between True qi and *Xie* qi in a person's eyes... it's just that most of us don't know it or acknowledge it.

General Demeanor

The person may look odd, like a cardboard cutout of themself, as if they were lost or out of sorts. In more extreme cases, they may even have a zombie-like look.

Accessibility Assessment

A diagnostic question you can ask the client is: Are you accessible to yourself?

This is a strange question to be asked and most people pause and seem confused at first. However, if the person actually has a Heart/*Yi* block, while they may look confused at first, they often do begin to understand, and respond with an answer like, "No, I don't think so, even though I don't know what that means."

What is Their Story?

It's important to have the client go back in their life story, if possible, to a time before they began to feel different or odd. What precipitated their illness or the change in their life?

Whenever a person's story has any of the following characteristics, the person may benefit from a Ghost Points treatment:

- A sudden change in their persona after a specific event that they can easily recount, such as an accident.
- A trauma history of any type. It's best not to go through the entire story in the assessment because you want them to tell the story during the treatment when the points are being activated.
- A description of having felt out of place or different from birth. The trauma may have been at birth or from unknown ancestral trauma.
- A story of ancestral trauma.
- Being told in childhood that they were wrong or bad or should be more like a parent or caregiver, in other words, if they were told to be someone they were not
- A story of an oppressive upbringing or abusive relationship.

The return to the root is peace. Peace: to accept what must be, to know what endures. In that knowledge is wisdom. Without it, ruin, disorder.

—Lao Tzu[10]

---

10 Lao Tzu, *Tao Te Ching: A Book about the Way and the Power of the Way*, trans. Ursula K. Le Guin (Boulder, CO: Shambala, 1998), 22.

Chapter Seven: The Ode of the Thirteen Ghost Points

Sun SiMiao's famous *Ode of the Thirteen Ghost Points* appears in several ancient texts. The version that has most influenced us is a poetic one that Leta has known and taught for the past twenty years. Unfortunately, despite extensive research, we have been unable to identify that version's translator.

As a result, we have taken all our learning, reviewed the various translations available to us, and compiled our own interpretive rendition of the Ode, which we include below. You may also wish to review another English translation in the book: *The Great Compendium of Acupuncture and Moxibustion Volume* IX, translated by Lorraine Wilcox.[11]

We have had the gift of numerous lectures with Master Jeffrey Yuen for over two decades, where he has explained the Ode to us in great detail. We are profoundly grateful for his invaluable teaching and believe that his generosity of spirit has helped us grow as students of Alchemy.

We are not experts in Sinology, nor are we fluent in Chinese. As with any translation from Chinese to English, interpretations can vary greatly and are often shaped by the era in which the translator lives. Many Chinese words can map to multiple English meanings. Despite our limited knowledge of the language, we have relied on our intuition, followed our inspiration, and drawn upon our experiences to create this translation.

---

[11] Yang Jizhou, *The Great Compendium of Acupuncture and Moxibusion: Zhen Jiu Da Cheng*, trans. Lorraine Wilcox (Portland, Oregon: The Chinese Medicine Database, 2011) 105-107.

Our "Ode" to the Ode of the Thirteen Ghost Points

For madness that arises from dark forces
The Thirteen Ghost points you must keep in mind!
Ghost Palace is the first point you must know,
Ghost Convincing is the next point to find.

All thirteen points will respond
Needle just one point at a time.
For bilateral points, left first for those who are more yang,
Right first for more yin beings will be sublime.

Needle Ghost Palace, Du 26, first
'Til the needle comes to rest.
Standing on the left to go in,
Removing from the right is best.[12]

The second point is Ghost Convincing, Lung 11,
Sitting below the thumb nail
Seeking the patient's true qi
With a 3-fen depth, success should prevail.

Hidden below the big toe nail,
Ghost Eyes, Spleen 1, it clears the vision
Two fen of needle's depth
Tears down Ghost's Fortress with certain precision.

---

[12] The original can be interpreted a number of ways. Is the needle inserted obliquely from the left (for males) and removed from the right side and vice versa for females? Or is this indicating that the entire set of needles are inserted according to gender and removed in reverse order (last in, first out) but with the practitioner standing on the opposite side of the body? In practice, we recommend the last in, first out when needle retention is being used.

Da Ling is the 4th point to seek
Sitting in the crease of wrist.
Needle five fen down
Clears the Ghost's Heart mist.

With a Fire needle warmed on Bladder 62
Along the Ghost Road is next to travel
Three times seven quick flashes
Causes the Ghost to unravel.

The sixth point's location
Far above Du 14 is best,
One cun into the hair, Ghost Pillow, Du 16,
Will bring some much needed rest.

Somewhere five fen below the ear lobe it sits,
The mystery lies in the Ghost Bed,
Using a warm needle
With a quick prick, it is bled.

Talking when you needle is a secret
Of Ren 24, the eighth point, Ghost Market
Insert going to the left side first
Removing from the right is the target.

Ghost Cave, the ninth point well on your journey
To continue expressing the sad heart song
You must venture into the palm line
You can call this point Lao Gong.

Du 23 is the tenth point to find
Quietly walk into the intimate Ghost Hall
The head's pinnacle point is the nearest to heaven,
Shang Xing is the name you may simply recall.

The eleventh point's Ghost is Hidden far from the eyes
Located at Ren 1 only for the men
Three moxa cones reveals the truth where it lies
The extra point on women is called Yu Men.

Wielding a Fire Mountain needle on Large Intestine 11
Find the twelfth point, called Ghost Official
Insert three sets of seven times rapidly
Releasing the Ghost's oppression is most beneficial.

Breaking the Ghost Seal is last to untie
Aim for the center of the bottom of the tongue
This extra point is simply called Gui Feng
Sending away the very last Ghost and now you're done.

For the bilateral points you find in the body
Needle both left and right sides
For points on the center line
Insert once where the Ghost point hides.

This ode to our esteemed teacher's legacy is honored by us here
This ancient path exists for those who do not fear
For all ghosts will find their way home
With the thirteen Ghost points ritual and your heart sincere.

The Ode of the Thirteen Ghost Points

男從左起針,女從右起針

第一針人中，名鬼宮 從左邊下針右邊出

第二針手大指爪甲下，名鬼信 入肉三分

第三針足大指爪甲下，名鬼壘 入肉二分

第四針掌後橫紋，名鬼心 入半寸（即太淵穴也)

第五針外踝下白肉際足太陽，名鬼路 火針七鋥，
鋥三下(即申 脈穴也)

第六針大椎上入髮際一寸，名鬼枕。火針七鋥，鋥三下

第七針耳前髮際宛宛中耳垂下五分，
名鬼床 火針七鋥，鋥三下

第八針承漿，名鬼市 從左出右

第九針手橫紋上三寸兩筋間，名鬼窟（即勞宮穴也)

第十針直鼻上入髮際一寸，名鬼堂。火針七鋥，鋥三下
(即上星穴也)

第十一針陰下縫，灸三壯，女人即玉門頭，名鬼藏

第十二針尺澤橫紋外頭接白肉際，名鬼臣 火針七鋥，
鋥三下（此即曲池)

第十三針舌頭一寸，當舌中下縫，刺貫出舌上，
名鬼封 仍以一板橫口吻，安針頭，令舌不得動

已前若是手足皆相對，針兩穴 若是孤穴，即單針之

At the crucial moment when the thirteen ponts have all been inserted, the physician should ask the patient which ghost or which demon made this disaster. The patient himself will tell the cause... When the patient has finished talking, the mania will stop.

—Zhen Jiu Da Cheng[13]

---

[13] Yang Jizhou, *The Great Compendium of Acupuncture and Moxibusion: Zhen Jiu Da Cheng*, trans. Lorraine Wilcox (Portland, Oregon: The Chinese Medicine Database, 2011) 108.

Chapter Eight: The Thirteen Ghost Points Treatment

With each Ghost Point, the goal is to access the True qi or the person's true nature. As we work with each point, the inauthentic qi begins to dissipate, allowing the release of stored trauma and negative life experiences from the body and mind, ultimately revealing the individual's authentic self.

The Void of the Heart: Heart Entrainment

We believe that the most effective way to access a person's True qi is from the void of your own heart. Why is this so? Inside your heart lies an empty space where the blood flows through—the dwelling space of your spirit or Shen. By focusing your attention on this space and extending the vibration from your *own* heart to the patient's heart, you create an extraordinary opportunity for transformation. This technique, which we call treating from the void of your heart, has proven to be the most powerful method for Ghost Point treatments. Stephen Harrod Buhner explains the science behind healing from the void of your heart in his *Secret Teachings of Plants* book.

> *When a person projects a heart-coherent field filled with caring, love and attention, living organisms respond to the information in the field by becoming more responsive, open, affectionate, animated, and closely connected...*

> *When these loving, practitioner-generated fields are detected and (naturally) amplified by ill people, healing rates of wounds are increased, pain decreases, hemoglobin levels shift, DNA alters, and new psychological states manifest.*[14]

In addition, if there are physical ghosts/*Gui* involved, communication with the *Gui* can also be done from the void of your heart.

Regardless of which of the Thirteen Ghost points you are working with, we recommend treating from the void of your heart. This approach is more important than a point location or needling technique and lies at the core of the cultivation of these points.

> *The void should not be frightening. Rather, it contains all possibilities.*[15]

The Heart Needs to Speak

Because this approach is so powerful, it's important that the practitioner cultivate not only the technique itself, but also ways to help a client through this level of transformative treatment, which in many cases requires the kind of deep rapport and professional intimacy we wrote about earlier.

One of the premises behind Alchemical work is that "the heart needs to speak." This means that when we're in pain, we may be refusing to speak about the pain. This avoidance of feelings or not even having access to the memories of what caused these feelings is common. In addition, the person may be of a more yin type and need more prompting to speak. Or if

---

[14] Stephen Harrod Buhner, The Secret Teachings of Plants: The Intelligence of the Heart in the Direct Perception of Nature (Rochester, VT: Bear & Company, 2004).

[15] Deng Ming-Dao, 365 *Tao: Daily Meditations* New York: HarperOne, 1992), 72.

a person is a more yang type, they may speak non-stop about surface-level topics as a type of avoidance of speaking about what's in the heart. In these cases, the practitioner may need to ask the person to take a break and listen internally for what comes up and what needs to be said.

The practitioner needs to cultivate their ability to be an instrument of the Divine in terms of gently guiding the conversation, learning how best to communicate without inserting themself into the treatment and affecting its outcome. At the same time, when the treatment is stalled, the practitioner needs to cultivate the knowledge and practice of how to bring up a topic or steer the conversation in the direction of what that person actually needs to talk about.

This is an art form, not a science, and for an effective treatment, the practitioner needs an advanced awareness of Five Element energetics in order to elegantly navigate the conversation with any of the five different elemental types.

Types of Treatments

Before jumping into working with the Ghost Points, you need to understand **how** to work with them.

Here are four examples of how the points can be incorporated into a treatment:

1. One or Two Points in a Single Treatment

When a client feels thwarted by life's challenges, a single Ghost Point or a combination of them may be the key to unlocking their path forward. By identifying the nature of their particular challenges you can then choose a corresponding point. For example, if you sense they have a lot of doubt, you could select Lung 11 (Ghost Convincing), which is targeted to help a person connect with their self-trust and the ability to step back onto their destiny's path.

Targeting the appropriate point can help dismantle the client's specific psychic and emotional blocks. A well-chosen Ghost Point can release repetitive thought loops and limiting beliefs, enabling a person to regain agency over their life's direction.

Case Study: Transformation from a Single Point

Leta once treated a woman with just a single point, which happened to be Ghost Market. The woman later shared how this one session profoundly changed her life. For years, she had struggled to speak positively about herself or share her talents with the world. This had hindered her career path and her relationships.

In the Thirteen Ghost Points treatment, Ghost Market is the point that unblocks self-expression. After being treated with just this one point, the woman found herself able to verbalize her worth. This shift enabled her to manifest major life changes.

Over the next year, this woman relocated to her dream city, landed her ideal job, and met her life partner. Where she had once felt creatively and romantically stifled, she now felt free and fulfilled.

According to her account, she believes and credits this one treatment for removing lifelong blocks around self-acceptance and assertion. By healing this root issue, other areas of her life effortlessly fell into alignment.

While one session may not always yield such dramatic results, this story demonstrates the holistic power of the Ghost Points. When the right point is selected at the right time to treat an imbalance, ripples of transformation can unfold in exciting and unexpected ways.

2. Working Through Some or All of the Points Over Time

If a person is experiencing more extensive emotional stagnation or blockage, then you can gradually work over time through all the Ghost Points in Trinities—the first twelve points broken down into groups of threes, with the thirteenth point often added to the fourth Trinity—to clear the emotional hooks. If they haven't had many traumatic events in life, a single Trinity or two Trinities (totaling six points) can sometimes be enough.

One note of caution: These points will bring up a lot of challenging experiences from the past. It can be difficult to progress slowly through these points when there's been significant past trauma. Multiple treatments may open old wounds for possibly extended periods between successive appointments. For this reason, in these types of cases it's often more beneficial to opt for doing all thirteen points in one extended session, which allows the person to walk through and release the painful memories and symptoms one after the other. However, sometimes releasing clients from a history of severe trauma does require longer periods of recovery between points. We will discuss this further on.

Case Study: Deep Betrayal Masked as Golfer's Elbow

Leta gradually worked through the Ghost Points over a long period of time with a man who was grappling with golfer's elbow. The pain was keeping him from playing golf and doing a number of other tasks. After many months of trying various physical approaches to healing his pain that yielded no results, we looked into potential emotional factors. He insisted that all was well in his life—he and his wife were happy, his kids were thriving, and he had no work-related stress. But because physical treatments weren't helping at all and despite his proclamations that he was emotionally feeling great, we decided to explore the Ghost Points treatment.

Over the course of a year, we slowly worked through the Thirteen Ghost Points, focusing on one or two each treatment. While he enjoyed the process, he didn't notice a shift in his pain until we reached Large Intestine 11, the 12th point, located at the end of the outer elbow crease. This point is associated with legal issues. To our surprise, the point opened a floodgate of stories about an employee embezzlement scheme involving a substantial portion of the client's life's savings. The employee was in the process of being tried with likely imprisonment looming. Because his employee was almost like a family member to him, the emotional betrayal on top of the financial threat was an especially hard blow. Remarkably, after addressing this specific point, the client's pain vanished completely, and did not return!

3. Doing the Trinity that Matches Where They Are

In some cases, it's possible to determine which subset of points (what we call trinities) is relevant to the client based on what symptoms they are experiencing. You would then do the First Trinity to open things up, followed by the Trinity you identified to address those particular symptoms.

4. Doing All Thirteen Points at Once: Long Sessions

If your client is facing significant emotional issues, physical challenges, or a trauma history, the full Thirteen Ghost Points protocol, as designed by Sun SiMiao, is the most comprehensive approach, covering all sorts of ill effects from trauma.

Drawing from two decades of extensive work with the Ghost Points, we've found that using the full set of points is remarkably effective in almost all cases. In fact, we typically lean towards working through the entire set with a person, while sometimes slightly tailoring our approach based on an individual's specific needs. This may be altered in the case of a history of severe trauma, however, which we discuss further on.

Our usual approach involves a single Ghost Points session of unlimited time—generally four to six hours—covering the entire set of thirteen points. This method gives individuals a clean slate by addressing all the potential ways that a person might have gotten hooked. It works to clear away any lingering issues and metaphorical skeletons in the client's closet.

The Thirteen Ghost Points are not randomly strung together. Following the sequence of the points is very important because they take a person on a journey from the most external, outward-facing part of them, which we call the Door to the Palace, through increasingly internal terrain, until they finally end up at the most internal part, which is their core identity.

So one of the many benefits of using all thirteen points in a single, long treatment is that if an early point in the sequence does not address the main issue the person is facing, it indicates that the issue is more likely rooted in a much deeper and more internal layer, such as guilt, shame, a lack of intimacy, or a feeling of oppression. Doing all thirteen points at once is a way to explore all the potential reasons that may be underlying the client's issues.

Ghost Point "Non-Needling Technique"

Whenever we treat a ghost point, we are attempting to access a person's True qi, which is called the *Zheng* qi or Authentic qi in Chinese Medicine. The point may have *Xie* qi or Evil/Inauthentic qi in it, and once that has been cleared, you can access the Authentic qi.

For this reason, acupuncturists have traditionally used a vibrating needle technique with the Ghost Points to disrupt and break up old patterns and to evoke change. The vibrating technique is the key to all Alchemical treatments.

While the Ghost Points can be needled with actual needles, we promote using a "non-needle" technique, which is an energetic form of acupressure that we call the "Energetic Approach" later in this chapter. Instead of inserting a needle into the point and vibrating it, we place a finger on the point and gently vibrate it, almost imperceptibly, on the surface of the skin. While the shaking seems minimal on the surface, it's quite intense internally, almost like a wave of energy rippling under the surface. Even our acupuncture students use this non-needle technique for many reasons.

In this book, we reference the traditional needling depth for each point so that when you use the non-needling technique, you can understand how deep your energetic focus should go.

> *Unless otherwise noted in this book, you can assume the vibrating technique is to be used with each point.*

Using All Thirteen Points Over Time for Severe Trauma

As we said earlier, another option for working with the points in the case of severe trauma is to work through the entire series of thirteen points but more slowly, over time. This is helpful if the person has had an extensive trauma history. In this case, it's unrealistic to expect everything to shift all at once. This type of work may take up to a year to bring about substantial changes, and it may make sense to consider focusing on only one ghost point during each treatment. In this case you might spend quite a long time on a single point, even up to an hour or more. This gradual and unhurried approach gives a person with an extensive trauma background the time they need to let go in a way that feels safe to them. It also allows for a new way of living life to emerge as it slowly reduces levels of extreme fear.

After the Treatment – Breaking Free from Old Habits and Patterns

Many people often feel a big shift after a treatment, but entrenched habits simply don't fade overnight. It can take three to six months for a person to release those habits once they recognize that those patterns no longer serve them. Those habits, rooted in fear and mistrust, were initially formed to protect the person against recurring negative experiences, with the resulting effect of essentially keeping them in a state of feeling "not free." Breaking free from these habits is a gradual process. Following the Ghost Point treatment, we often encourage our clients to practice self-forgiveness and more particularly pay attention to their thoughts and activities in their daily lives. It's common for them to express realizations like, "I've come to understand that I no longer need to approach things in that way."

Case study: Sudden Unexplained Smoking-Cessation

One example of this kind of transformation was a female client who returned to the clinic two months after her Ghost Point treatment and said, "Guess what? I just stopped smoking the other day."

This was surprising since she hadn't previously declared that she wanted to stop smoking or that she was even a smoker at all.

When asked if she had been trying to quit for a long time, she replied, "No, not really. I mean, I'm happy I'm not smoking anymore and know it's better that way for me, but I wasn't intentionally trying to stop. After the Ghost Points treatment, I realized I just didn't need to smoke anymore. I lost the desire or the need to smoke, I guess."

Classical Indications

Throughout this chapter, the signs and symptoms we've included for each Ghost Point are a blend of our personal observations and the classical symptoms, carefully selected from various sources, especially the teachings of Master Jeffrey Yuen over the past two decades. If you're not dealing with severe mental illness, many of the traditionally attributed signs and symptoms are quite rare. We've included them here as a reference for those interested in that specialized area of practice.

The First Trinity of Ghost Points – How You Interface with the World

The First Trinity of Ghost Points addresses how a person interacts with the world on a day-to-day basis. It can reveal how people get hooked into patterns that make them live inauthentically. When these pesky hooks persist over a long period of time, they can change a person more deeply, which signifies that a person may also need additional Ghost Point Trinities.

Often the First Trinity represents how you respond to trauma. We respond to trauma physically, emotionally, and spiritually. Trauma can create physical patterns on the cellular level that are very difficult to access intellectually or even through talk therapy. We might also have emotional/spiritual effects, such as panic attacks and other Post Traumatic Stress Disorder (PTSD) symptoms, like sweating and hyperventilating that seem illogical but result from triggers stemming from past trauma that appear in our current environment. Modern medicine tries to address this with medication, but in many cases it appears that the medicine doesn't address the root cause.

The first point represents the door to you. If the door isn't operating correctly, it allows the ghost to enter into you.

Then the ghost needs to find a way to hook into you, which leads to the second point. If the ghost can convince you that it is supposed to be there or that it was always meant to be there, it's not naturally expelled by your system as it should be.

Then the next layer down occurs when it sets up its home within you. The third point represents how the ghost sets up its home within you when it manages to stick around long enough. It then begins to influence the way you perceive the world, in order to build a case for why it should stay. It needs to prove to you that it's supposed to be there, or at least why it makes sense that you're stuck with it being there. It looks for evidence in the world around you to reinforce the idea that it should remain firmly embedded in you. This prompts a shift in how you view yourself and the world, forcing you to undergo changes based on its influence over you.

In Chinese Medicine, these first three points are all points for resuscitation. Choosing to use them indicates that you are trying to reconnect with your True qi, or your true nature, so that you can cast out the "ghost" by being more fully yourself. If you can fully embody yourself, there will be no more room for the "ghost."

The first three points are also a trinity of Heaven, Humanity, and Earth: One point is on the head for Heaven, one on the hands for Humanity, and one on the foot for Earth.

We believe that Sun SiMiao likely selected these as the first three points on the head, hands, and feet due to their particular ability to clear phlegm. At the time, it was believed that there were four types of phlegm:

- *Yi Yin* or fluid phlegm – which translates as diffused fluid and refers to flooding of fluids in the body, causing edema and swellings
- *Zhi Yin* or limbic phlegm – which is cold congested fluid, causing poor posture (can't stand up straight), dizziness, or wobbliness (even feeling faint)
- *Xuan Yin* – which means suspended fluid and refers to a feeling of being pressed down, causing chest oppression and difficulty breathing
- *Tan Yin* – which means phlegm fluid, and refers to the expectoration of a lot of phlegm and sputum as well as having confusion from phlegm "misting the mind"

It was believed that these different types of phlegm could affect the head, chest, and limbs. Sun SiMiao may have selected Lung 11 to disperse phlegm from the chest and move it up and out to the four limbs. And the Spleen 1 point may have been selected because the Spleen governs the four limbs.

The theory at the time, postulated by Chao Yuanfang in his book *General Treatise on Causes and Manifestations of All*

Diseases, was that phlegm is created by the Spleen, and the Lung tries to break it up and cough it out. Because the *Jing*/ Well points release to the exterior and open the sensory portals, he may have selected these points on the Lung and Spleen channels to purify the system of any phlegm or worms/ parasites.

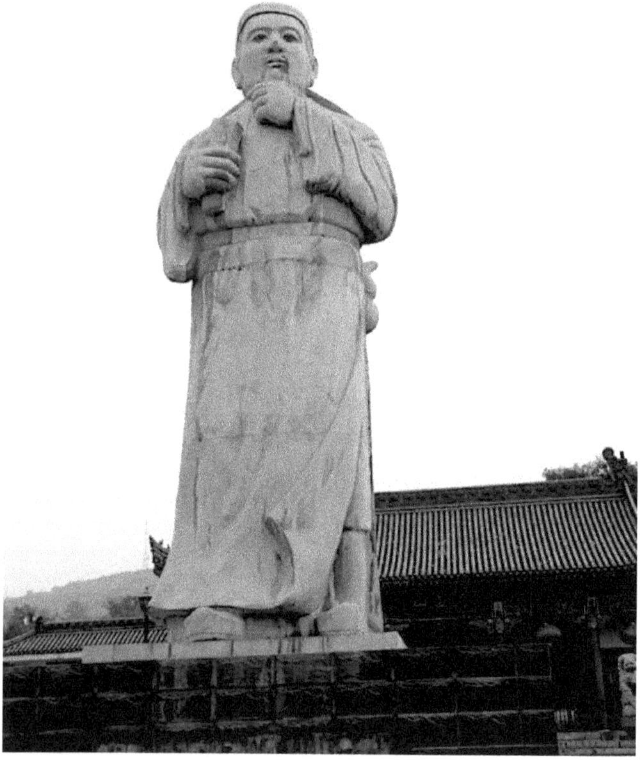

Sun SiMaio, from the base of his home, Hunan, China

1 Ghost Palace – Gui Gong, Du 26

The initial point, known as Ghost Palace, symbolizes the doorway or the grand entrance to your palace. Your palace is your body/mind/spirit. The ghost has entered your palace as a guest but is going to try to stay and make a home in your body.

Located just below the nose and above your mouth, in the area known as the philtrum, the point sits between two important gateways that interface between you and the outside world in the center of the main sensory orifices—your mouth and nose. This location is crucial for absorbing the essential sustenance necessary for your survival—both the food you consume and the air you breathe.

The questions here are: How does this doorway or "door to you" actually operate? Does the door to your true self operate in harmony with your authentic nature? Does it open and close appropriately as needed?

Perhaps your door naturally swings wide open, welcoming everyone to join your life and your festivities without the need for a fancy invite. This may be how you generally interact with the world, like an extrovert, or what we would call a more yang person.

For example, you may love to host parties at your house and have no qualms about receiving uninvited guests who want to crash the party. Your motto might be: "The more the merrier!"

However, what if someone comes into your palace and causes trouble? If that were to happen, you might start acting a bit more cautious and discerning about who gets VIP access to your inner sanctum. You might even station a metaphorical bouncer at your door to keep out those less-than-welcome guests.

Life's disappointing and painful experiences might even make you think about shutting that door entirely, or perhaps just leaving a peephole there, for you to look out and keep an eye on the outside world.

Or maybe you're a person who naturally cherishes quiet moments of reflection and appreciates a bit of privacy. In that case, your natural inclination might be having a door that's just slightly ajar or maybe even closed most of the time with only a tiny peephole. You might naturally lean towards being more selective about who and how many people you allow into your space—definitely not the type with a crowded house party vibe.

If this sounds like you, you might be authentically more yin by nature, meaning you're more of an introvert than an extrovert.

However, if you have experienced distressing events in life, you may feel the urge to add many more locks and barricades on the door. Even with those in place, you may feel the need to keep a vigilant eye on that door. This can be very taxing and exhausting when it happens day in and day out.

In another challenging scenario, your door may have been damaged or blown off entirely by a past trauma, leaving you feeling defenseless as the outside world floods into your inner sanctum and you feel powerless to stop it.

These types of situations can lead to your door functioning in ways that don't align with your true self, and this misalignment will be unique to each person. In some cases, you might no longer feel free to express yourself authentically. Trauma and negative experiences may have caused you to change how you perceive and welcome the outside world.

Then the question becomes: How "should" your door operate? The word "should" raises a valid point to be considered. Every person is unique, with unique experiences and a unique journey. Because of this, we feel that each person is entitled to explore their own life path and decide what is the happiest and most fulfilling life they want to live. There can be many ways for a door to operate.

Unwanted Guests – Who Do You Let in Your Doors?

What actually happens when something or someone energetically enters through your door that doesn't align with your true self? Typically, most people can shrug it off effortlessly without much thought or energy. They promptly dismiss and expel anything that doesn't resonate with them, refusing to let it linger. They simply let it go.

Take the example of when Leta was in the Peace Corps in West Africa many years ago. Her group of 30 people shared every meal together. One day, the group must have consumed tainted food. Most of the members instinctively headed to the bathroom, purging everything that didn't align with their well-being either through vomiting or diarrhea. Then the sickness eventually passed, leaving them feeling better and onto the fast track of recovery.

However, a small minority of the group actually ended up quite ill, needing medicine to combat bacteria or parasites and were eventually sent home.

What was different about the ones who got sick? Why did they fall ill when the majority didn't? We think the Ghost Points can provide an explanation or a theory that can explain many such examples, not just this one. The people who couldn't recover may have had an opening or a doorway for the disease to get in and then stay in.

Where did this opening come from? It could have been an on-going belief that foods can cause such illnesses, creating an underlying constant fear of eating bad food. Or some may have believed that they had a weak stomach and couldn't handle tainted food in general. Perhaps they believed that their whole family line was genetically sensitive, and so they carried embedded in them the idea that "we always get sick."

In any of these cases, the body will then fail to expel the food that isn't in alignment with the digestive system, and then when they do get sick, it further confirms the original belief system.

For individuals who get really sick, like the ones in Leta's story, the next Ghost Point to be activated would be Ghost Convincing. We will fully explain the Ghost Convincing point later, but it's helpful to know a bit about how it affected those Peace Corps folks. The people who became ill began to believe that the illness was there to stay, and there was nothing they could do about it. They became "convinced" of something that wasn't true to them. If they had truly been in alignment with their authentic selves, they would not have actually become ill because **illness is never the natural state of authentic qi**.

On the other hand, the "ghost" that enters the Palace doesn't have to be something coming from outside the person, as in that story when people ingested tainted food (which we call *Gu*/worms) or when there is an invasion from some entity (*Gui*/ghost) or even by an Elemental/Climatic energy like Heat or Wind.

In many cases, the "ghost" is a thought form the person created. This is often what can occur after a traumatic event. The human mind tries to rationalize what happened and come up with a new way of being that attempts to keep the person safe, to ensure that the trauma will never occur again. In this case, the person can become possessed by their own mind, which just means that the thoughts the mind created aren't true to that person. For example, a person may come up with the thought that "I am an inherently bad person, and that's why these bad things keep happening to me." This would be a form of "possession."

In this context, the Ghost Palace point represents the initial reaction to the trauma or the entering of the negative or obsessive thought forms into the mind.

We know that illnesses can stem from external pathogens, like viruses, parasites, and bacteria, but why is it that some people's acute conditions turn into chronic, persistent conditions like long-COVID, chronic Lyme disease, or antibiotic-resistant staph infections, such as MRSA?

The answer to this question lies in the person's mindset, often based on past-life experiences. The person may have had a strong conscious or unconscious belief that they were fundamentally not healthy and had a weak constitution. So their immune system was depressed by this "possessing" thought form, and thus, the external pathogen wasn't eliminated. That belief is continuing to operate in their current life. Whether the idea came from a past life or this current life, it can be a "which came first, the chicken or the egg?" situation. Was the weakened immune system caused by the negative thought forms? Or were the negative thought forms caused by the weakened immune system? After doing the Thirteen Ghost Points now for over twenty years, it's our belief that in a large majority of the people we've worked with who had health issues, the body was initially responding to negative thought forms, often caused by trauma and negative events or situations in the person's life, such as internalizing the negativity of their parents when they were young.

More than "Just" Health Palace Concerns

The Ghost Palace point applies to other types of life situations that are related to the other Nine Palaces, not just the Health Palace. For example, a person might have received negative feedback at some point in their workplace, and suddenly their Career Palace becomes problematic. Coworkers talk behind their back, they get passed over for promotions, or maybe they even get fired.

Or a mother might be thrilled about the arrival of a new baby; however, the baby ends up crying a lot, and the mother can't sleep. In the desperation caused by a lack of sleep, she begins to form negative opinions about the child, which then creates excessive worry about the child, which would be a Children/Creativity Palace issue that could go on for years.

Or a bad breakup could result in a lifetime of negative beliefs about the chances of finding healthy intimacy, thus making the Relationship Palace feel troubled and lonely.

The way you interact with the world is the key factor for this point. Thus, in a general sense, the Ghost Palace point can also be related to how you think others perceive you. For example, a person who harbors low self-esteem can end up being seen by others and the world at large as less than capable, even if it's not true.

Indications[16]

This point's signs and symptoms tend to be related to interactions with the outer world. For the most part, the symptoms tend to be rather mild and not very noticeable at first. The changes within the body can be quite subtle. But the person may feel or seem "off" and not be able to pinpoint anything specific.

Sensory organ symptoms: The "ghost" is challenging the way the person interacts with the world and is trying to control how the person senses the world, causing sensory symptoms related to the eyes, ears, nose, and mouth.

Spine stiffness: The body senses that something foreign has entered into it and needs to be expelled. We call this "Wind" in Chinese Medicine. This causes the yang qi, which runs along the spine (the ladder of life), to be activated, which can cause the spine to feel stiff.

PTSD-like symptoms: Post-traumatic stress may be causing panic attacks, shortness of breath, loss of appetite, feeling out of sorts, difficulty communicating, and a perception of negative voices in the head saying things like, "you're no good."

See the Classical Indications section on page 115 about signs and symptoms.

Treating Ghost Palace

When we treat the Ghost Palace point, we focus on healing the person's external, outward-facing self and how it engages with the outer world. The outer world may have been the original source of trauma in the past. If that is the case, the point may have a lot of disturbance that can feel like static. It's as if the point is a door to that static, which is taking place deep inside the body.

As we treat the point, we're feeling for that internal disturbance to clear or calm down until it feels peaceful. If the person is aware of their own energy or internal state, they may report feeling more relaxed inside. However, not all people have body awareness, so it's not imperative for the person to report a shift right away. Each person is unique.

This is the first point in the protocol because it can "summon and lift the yang qi." The body needs yang qi to push out anything that doesn't belong there.

Needle depth: 2–5 fen (.2 to .5 cun) or "until the needle comes to rest."[17]

Position of the practitioner: We recommend sitting behind the head of the client, looking toward the person's feet so that the treatment begins with less talking and less face-to-face interaction. You are not in a threatening position for their door/doorway in any way. Place one hand on the point and cradle the head with the other hand, or rest your other hand near the Du 20 area on the top of the head.

Some talking can be appropriate about the nature of the point, but it's good for the person to have a bit more space on this first point to get the feeling of what the treatment is doing internally. You can move to the side and face the person if more face-to-face talking is required.

Needling: As with all the Ghost Points, a vibrational needling technique is used. Traditionally this point was

[17] It's unclear in Sun SiMiao's ode what the needle depth should be.

needled through the upper lip to the frenulum, but we do not recommend that for modern times and have not found it to be clinically necessary.

Energetic Approach: Place your finger on the point and feel the frenulum underneath. Imagine the energy of the point connecting with the frenulum beneath while vibrating gently.

Client Reactions: Activating this point may cause quivering in the body (sometimes the entire body) or nasal discharge.

Case Study: Angry Father

One woman didn't think she'd had any serious trauma in her life except that she shared the fact that she had grown up with an angry father. However, she also explained that she did not feel angry inside herself but instead felt that he was the angry one. Yet, somehow this anger in childhood had shut her door. She was a Fire Element Energetic type, and she wanted to be very open and social in life, but she just wasn't able to open her doorway to the world.

During the treatment, this point was very activated, what we would describe as being intensely on guard. We spent over an hour working with this one point because this was where a lot of her trauma was. If it wasn't safe to open her door at home, it certainly didn't feel safe to open it out in the world.

After the treatment, she began to engage with the world in a wholly new and joyful way. She also began to develop more long-lasting relationships. Something had shifted in the way she received newcomers into her life. She released the fear of anger in herself and was free to be more open and loving.

Ghost Palace: Self-Cultivation

You can cultivate this point either as a meditation (see below) or as a journaling exercise or both.

Cultivating this point is a process of finding the most authentic way to interact with the outer world. Working with this point allows you to return to a time when you engaged the world according to your true nature... whether you tend to be bolder, like an extrovert or more shy, like an introvert.

You can think about what feels most natural to you and how you may or may not be presenting a completely different "door" to the world.

To do this as a journaling exercise, think back over your entire life and try to determine which period of time was the happiest in your life, whether it's your current present time or a past joyful phase of your life. If you cannot remember a time that you ever felt happy, try to recall the time in your life that you felt the most content or the most at ease.

Remembering this time, contemplate how you interacted with the outer world. During these happier times, what was your door like and how did it operate specifically? Was the door wide open and welcoming to all or did you prefer to have a closed door that allowed you to evaluate who you wanted to interact with? What did it feel like to have ease and happiness in your life?

Now think about why this time in your life changed. Did an event, job, or person trigger something in you that changed the way you interacted with the world? Compare that to your current life interactions and beliefs, and ask yourself how you have changed since then.

Answer these questions to guide you toward making changes in your life. What adjustments would you need to make in order to express your most authentic self in the way you engage with the world? Can you realign and be your truest self when you interact with others?

The Ghost Palace Meditation

The purpose of this meditation is to discover the true essence of the door to your Palace, enabling a deeper understanding of how you can more genuinely connect with the world around you.

This meditation draws upon your ability to visualize, but if you're not particularly visual, you can engage more with the feelings or sounds involved. Feel free to incorporate all your senses into this exercise.

You can begin by finding a quiet space and having your journal or notebook next to you for recording your reflections after the meditation. Then follow the Relax Your Body and Clear Your Mind Meditation on page 54 of this book. You can listen to the free guided version at the Alchemy Learning Center (AlchemyLearningCenter.com).

Once you are relaxed, take a few moments to clear your mind of any thoughts that arise. Now you are ready to start the Ghost Palace meditation.

Begin by revisiting a period in the past when life was positive, and you felt the most authentic in your life. If recalling this is challenging due to early-life trauma, simply focus on a time in your life that held the most positivity for you.

From the positive period of time you selected, when life was good, happy, and safe, envision a home (imaginary or real) that represents this period of your life, and picture the entrance to your home or palace, visualizing the door in any way that resonates with you.

Each person's authentic door will look and operate differently. For some, it may be wide open, while for others, it could be securely locked with nothing but a peephole. The crucial factor is not the type of door you have, but rather that it operates authentically, in alignment with your true nature.

What does the door to your home look like? What color is the door? What kind of landscape is it located in? Is it crafted from glass, wood, or metal? How thick is it? Does it look like it has a particular texture?

Now imagine how the door operates. Is the door wide open all the time? Is the door closed most of the time? Is it there to protect you or to allow for anyone to have access to you? Is the door locked and if so how many locks are on that door? Or is the door barely on its hinges or blown off?

How did you feel about the door when times were good? Did it feel like it was your true door, operating authentically the way your door needs to operate for you? Did it feel like it was your normal door when times were good?

Now let's come forward in time to the present time. How is your door in the world today? Does it look different?

Does it operate differently than the older door? If so, how does it feel different?

Perhaps your door, once wide open and inviting, is now closed and secured with many locks.

Maybe it used to be shut, and you had full control over it when it opened. But now, is that sense of control gone?

Was your door previously locked all the time with a small peephole and now the door has been completely blown off?

How does it operate for you now? How has that changed?

Take a few moments to think about the changes in your door.

When you are ready, open your eyes.

In your journal write about the true nature of your door and whether it's current state is your authentic door. If your door is not operating authentically now, what would the true nature of your door be like? You can listen to a guided version of this meditation at the Alchemy Learning Center (AlchemyLearningCenter.com).

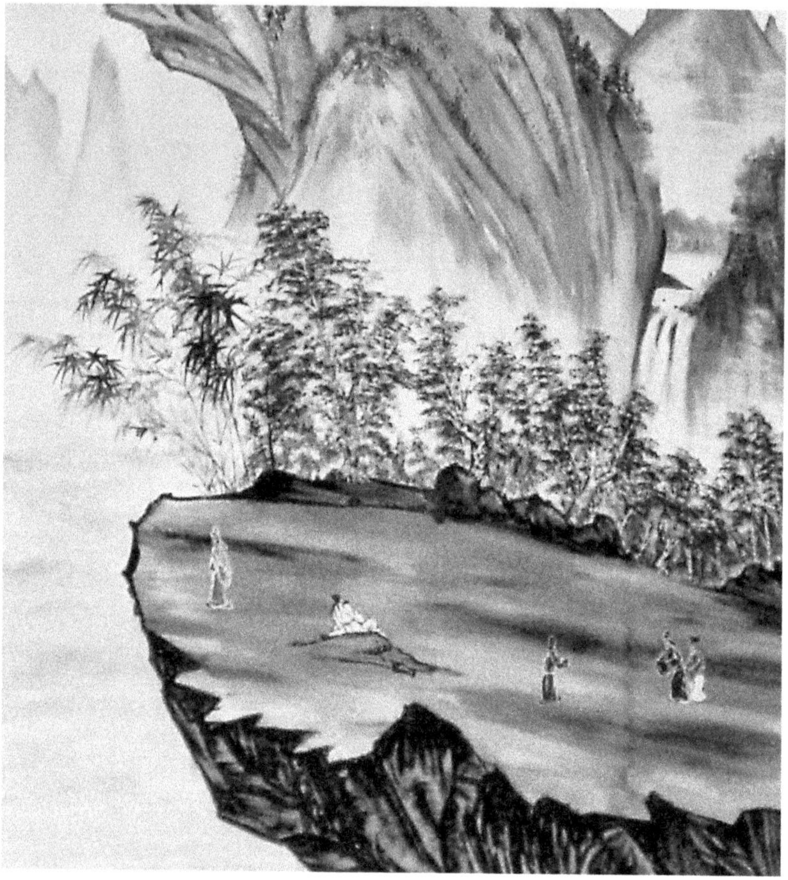

Painting from temple wall at the home of Sun SiMiao, Hunan, China

2 Ghost Convincing/Faith/Trust – *Gui Xin*, Lung 11

Consider the countless times in life where external influences or negative experiences have somehow convinced you to allow something undesirable into your world. Allowing these unwelcome elements to persist in your life ends up thwarting your true nature and disrupting your inner harmony. These unwanted experiences can come in all sizes from extra small all the way to extra large.

The second Ghost Point, known as Ghost Convincing, shows us what happens when something gets into you that doesn't align with your authentic self. When negativity or the "ghost" finds its way in, how does it gain your trust? How do you handle it? Do you throw it out? Or do you get convinced it's okay if it stays? Or maybe you believe you're too powerless to expunge it and that it's too strong to be dispelled, which leaves you trapped in the situation.

When you become convinced that something inauthentic has entered your life, it can lead to an erosion of self-trust. This loss of trust may manifest in two ways: either you begin to question your capacity to accurately discern what's right for you, or you start doubting your ability to keep what doesn't serve you at bay.

The Ghost Convincing point works by addressing and rectifying these influences in order to provide a realignment with your truth. This realignment not only aids in breaking free from the grip of undesirable influences but also enables you to discern what truly resonates with you so that you can feel empowered to navigate your life with greater resilience.

Indications

This point's signs and symptoms tend to be related to the way a person doubts their own beliefs based on outer world opinions and influences. For the most part, the symptoms are fairly mild and not very noticeable at first. The changes within the body are subtle. But the person may feel or seem "off" and not be able to pinpoint anything specific.

Voice change: The person's voice can start to sound different. For example, sometimes a voice may sound very young, almost childlike, in a way that doesn't match the person's age at all.

Indifference: The person may feel indifferent to the world around them due to the fact that their sensory orifices (which are their doorways to the world) are now being controlled by the "ghost." This means they are no longer receiving trustworthy input from their senses. They may even have phlegm clogging the orifices (eyes, nasal passages, ears, and throat).

Hearing voices: The negative self-talk may be more intense than it was with the Ghost Palace point, due to the self-doubt. The voices or even high-pitched sounds may seem to be coming from outside the person, similar to tinnitus.

Throat *Bi* (Painful) Obstruction: The person may find it difficult to speak their truth, as if their throat is closed, or they have a strange sore throat with some heat-related symptoms and pain.

Treating Ghost Convincing

When we treat Ghost Convincing, our goal is to find the kernel of authenticity residing deep within each person, a source or truth that they can tap into. Often, individuals have become disconnected from this profound inner knowing, what we call Trust with a Capital T. Being convinced over and over again to disregard their inner Trust has fostered significant self-doubt, clouding their judgment, making life in general very challenging to navigate with clarity and confidence.

This is a *Jing*-Well point, located near the nail bed of the thumb. The *Jing*-Well points are useful for opening up portals/ orifices (such as the eyes, ears, nose, and mouth) to release pathogens or anything that is not true to a person, like a "ghost."

In particular, Lung 11 has an effect on the tongue, in the sense that it improves communication by "opening the tongue." It also opens the Lungs for increased breathing capacity (if the person has shortness of breath) and releases any phlegm in the Lungs.

This point can also treat tinnitus, thus targeting any voices the person is hearing. It is important to allow the person to voice any of the negative messages they may be playing over and over again in their head in order to uncover the inherent truth that lies beneath their negativity.

Needling: 3 fen (.3 cun) Use a vibrational needling technique. Sun SiMiao's Ode states that this point should be needled 3 fen (which is normally needled shallowly—no more than 1 fen—or bled).

Because we use and teach our students to use non-needle techniques, we don't have experience with actually needling this point to this depth. We have read of practitioners using the flying needle technique instead (flicking the needle upon insertion), perhaps to avoid using the prescribed needle depth, which may be quite painful for the patient. However, we have no clinical experience with the flying needle technique.

Energetic Approach: Use your fingernail to find the dip at the base of the Lung 11 nail bed. It is a very small area for the tip of your finger to fit into, so you can imagine that your finger is a needle and focus your energy into the point (3 fen) while vibrating. Then place your attention internally on the person's core truth. Most of our acupuncture students opt to use this technique rather than using the actual needles.

Moxibustion: We typically find that this point doesn't need moxibustion except in cases where the point doesn't seem to be shifting after some time. However, you can add moxibustion to help create enough yang heat to purge the ghost. Moxibustion on this point opens the throat to help clear any phlegm from the chest or discharge it from the nose if there is lingering dampness. It's also useful for nosebleeds.

Ghost Convincing Self-Cultivation

Like all of us, you were born with an innate knowing, even as you continue to learn the ways of the world. This pillar of internal strength and individuality is something that fuels your sense of self-trust. The world may not agree with your truth, but if it's *your* truth, you can still completely trust that truth.

At times, though, you may lose your confidence and allow doubt to set in. Cultivating the Ghost Convincing point allows you to rediscover and fortify your self-belief, almost as if you're reconnecting your umbilical cord back to the Divine. It's an unshakable trust in what you feel and know to be true.

Ultimately it's a trust in the Divine and your connection to it that allows you to be genuine and authentic. From that sincere, whole-hearted place, you can more easily confront and overcome challenges that might otherwise shake your confidence in your truth.

The Ghost Convincing point serves as a catalyst for seeking to rediscover and fortify your belief in yourself, reconnecting you to your self-trust, or what we like to call *Trust with a capital T.*

Once this reconnection is established, the point becomes a powerful ally in confronting and overcoming challenges without self-doubt clouding your decision-making process.

Ghost Convincing Meditation

The purpose of this meditation is to discover any lingering doubts that may be haunting you (like "Ghosts"). These doubts could stem from painful experiences, repetitive negative thoughts, or external influences that have taken root within you.

The goal is to help you reconnect with your innate ability to trust yourself.

You can begin by finding a quiet space and having your journal or notebook next to you for recording your reflections after the meditation. Then follow the *Relax Your Body and Clear Your Mind Meditation* on page 54 of this book. You can listen to the free guided version at the AlchemyLearningCenter.com. Now you are ready to start the Ghost Convincing meditation.

Begin by taking a moment to settle into your heart space, where your authentic self and true essence dwells. Within this space resides your personal truth, distinct from what others think and the social expectations they put on you. Your heart governs your own alignment and resonance with your life experiences. It can discern what feels true and in alignment with you and what feels false or out of alignment with you.

Take a comprehensive look at your life, both past and present. What in your life has deviated from your truth or currently doesn't resonate with your authentic self? It might involve a relationship you're trying to forge that is difficult, a health issue contradicting your true well-being, or a mental state filled with uncertainty. Explore the various ways that doubt may have infiltrated your life—whether it's one or two specific areas or multiple aspects of your life.

Select one doubt that feels significant for you right now and sit with it for a moment. Think back to when this doubt first entered your consciousness. What happened that made you doubt your truth? What new belief or beliefs did you adopt that led to a change in your convictions?

If you had always believed you were healthy, what were the first ideas in your mind that convinced you that you weren't healthy? If you grew up with a sense of abundance, what thoughts initially contributed to a feeling of scarcity or an inability to connect with your wealth? If you perceived yourself as lovable, what factors led to feelings of being unlovable? If you felt connected to the Divine, what convinced you that you were no longer connected or supported by the universe?

Whatever had been true to you, what convinced you to begin to doubt that?

Now return to your heart space, where you can establish a connection with your truth, the genuine essence of who you are. Examine what aspects of this doubt do not align with your authenticity. Is the label you've been giving yourself truly reflective of your true essence?

Challenge yourself to consider the opposite of this doubt. For example, if you doubt your health and have felt unhealthy, explore the idea of being fundamentally healthy. Does that resonate within you, even if pain or discomfort in your body in the current reality is trying to make you think otherwise?

Regardless of the nature of the doubt, reconnect with its opposite and find a pathway that leads you to your truth. Immerse yourself in your authentic truth.

When you are ready, you can open your eyes.

Now take a moment and in your journal, write down the characteristics associated with the doubt and the emotions that surfaced when you reconnected with your truth. You can listen to a guided version of this meditation at the Alchemy Learning Center (AlchemyLearningCenter.com).

Case Studies: Feeling Dumb and Dumber

A number of clients we have seen in the clinic over the years had been told as children that they were not smart, when they clearly were. One client's mother said, "Book learning is not for you," and as a result, she didn't go to college, even though her parents, aunts, and uncles all did. Instead she got married and had children, which was fine with her. But that fact hadn't kept her from always feeling "less than," even though she was quite smart. This feeling had influenced her all through her life, making her feel unsure of herself whenever she tried to assert her opinions in any way.

In this case, being told by a parent that she lacked intelligence profoundly impacted her identity and shook her belief in her sense of self. While working with this point, she came to realize that she'd always possessed intelligence. In fact, she began to understand that she happened to be quite brilliant, and it was her mother's insecurities about her own intelligence that led her to criticize her daughter. This point helped her to reestablish a connection with a deeper sense of knowing and wisdom, far surpassing what she had ever before been able to acknowledge within herself. Following the treatment, her faith in her own intelligence was rejuvenated.

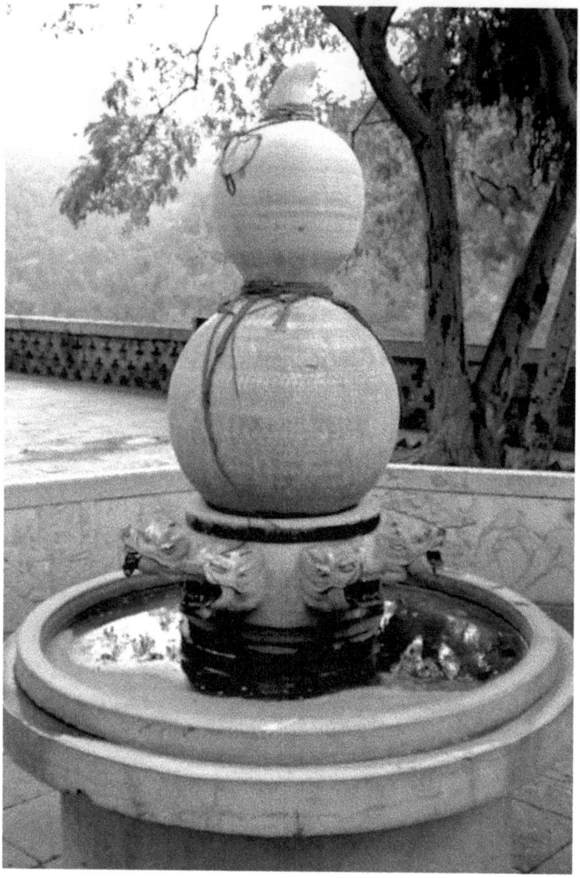

Healer's Gourd statue at home of Sun SiMiao, Hunan, China

3 Ghost Eyes/Ghost Fortress – *Gui Lei*, Spleen 1

At this point the "ghost" is moving inwards and also gaining control over the limbs. As a result, the person begins doing what the ghost wants them to do. This point is an Earth point. By moving into Earth, the ghost has begun to affect the person's *Jing*/Essences. It is also the transition between the first and second trinities and a good one for that purpose, since it's a connector to the next point Pericardium 7, which is the Earth point in Fire.

Once something gets hooked into you and you become convinced that it's here to stay, your perspective on the world becomes skewed. You no longer see the world the same way. In fact, it's as if you were wearing different colored lenses when you look out on the world. You start to see evidence that supports whatever you were *convinced* about.

For example, if you once contract an intestinal bacteria, you might thereafter become wary of every meal you eat. As you sit down to eat, you might vigilantly scrutinize your food, noting imperfections that others might overlook. After a meal, you might be acutely aware of any unusual sensations in your stomach, almost anticipating running to the bathroom. If you have had Lyme disease, you may think that a tick will find you every time you go out into nature, thereby making you want to stay inside most of the time where you feel safer.

In these cases, the "hook" has deeply embedded itself in you. You are no longer free to see the world as it really is. You start fabricating reasons to support your new convictions.

Consider how many times witnesses to the same event recount distinctly different stories. Each observer interprets the event through their unique perspective, as if they were wearing different colored lenses. If any of these witnesses had experienced a similar event in the past, their interpretation of the recent event may be colored by those previous experiences. As a result, they might see "evidence" of the beliefs they formed based on those earlier experiences, while another witness might report an entirely different narrative.

This is an example of how our sight, specifically how we see the world, gets subverted by a "ghost" or emotional hook.

Once our eyes are looking for and compiling evidence to support our doubts, then we begin to build a fortress with this evidence. The fortress is built out of the stories of the past that fortify the ghost's existence. The stories are based on a single viewpoint. If an earthquake could come and shake up the foundation of the fortress, the walls might come tumbling down.

The "ghost" lives behind the fortress and is protected by all the evidence you see that supports the ghost's existence. This fortress becomes bolstered by years of watching for and collecting more and more evidence that supports the "ghost's" arguments.

Indications

Ghost Eyes/Ghost Fortress' signs and symptoms are starting to inhabit a slightly deeper space as the "ghost" begins to take over perception and build the fortress inside.

Eyes: The person's eyes may seem disengaged because their *Shen* is not present in them. Or their eyes may seem glassy or shiny due to leakage of qi. In cases of actual possession, it's at this point that we can potentially see evidence of the "ghost" in the person's eyes. This could be the lack of light in the eyes or a seeming additional presence in the eyes. This can show up very differently in each person, but might be described as a shifting or vibrating in some cases.

Dreams: The person dreams of very yin places, like water or graveyards, and there is often tossing and turning at night.

Heat: An increase in heat in the body may cause excessive fantasizing, explosive emotional outbreaks including screaming or raving if pushed too much, or even destructive behaviors prompted by the voices in the person's head. There may also be physical manifestations such as hemorrhoids or heavy menstrual blood due to the accumulation of yin.

Chest Oppression: The person may feel as if they have a cinder block sitting on their chest or feel like they're being held down.

Dampness: The person may feel confused, foggy, disoriented, depressed, fearful, anxious, disgusted with the world, reclusive, withdrawn, or disconnected from friends and family. The person may appear comatose or have slowed down speech, abdominal fullness or distention, or a loss of appetite. They may even hear voices in their head saying, "You don't need anyone, and no one cares about you".

Numbness: The "ghost" is now affecting the hands and feet, which may feel cold or numb, requiring that the *Jing*-Well points be used in this protocol.

Treating Ghost Eyes

The Ghost Eyes point works to eliminate those strange tinted lenses from a person's eyes, enabling them to see the unfolding events of their life with clarity. *Jing*-Well points open the portals of perception in order to facilitate the release of pathogens, and in this case, the pathogen is this strange pattern of seeing things through a skewed "ghost" lens.

Once the eyes are cleared in this way, they'll no longer need to be on constant alert for the recurrence of negative events. In other words, the post-traumatic stress pattern that has kept them perpetually on guard against repeat traumas can finally be at rest.

This means that the sentries they have set up on their fortress lookout towers that they'e built over time are no longer necessary to vigilantly watch for whatever bad things they expect to happen. However, as with all the Ghost Points, it's important to note that new "eyes" can take a little time to adjust to this new way of seeing... sometimes up to six months.

Needling: 2 fen (.2 cun) Use vibrating needle action or you can use the flying needle technique (flicking needle upon insertion) or the hot needle technique can be used to excite the energy.

Energetic Approach: If the ghost has established a fierce stronghold in the fortress, you may need to use more vigorous vibration with your finger on this point to create an energetic "earthquake."

Moxibustion: Moxibustion on *Jing*-Well points is effective to excite the energy. You can use moxa to clear dampness and confusion and to create yang heat to purge the ghost. Spleen 1 is more amenable to moxibustion than some other points that regulate blood.

Ghost Eyes Self-Cultivation

The constant vigilance of Ghost Eyes, always on the lookout for danger even in peaceful situations, can be quite draining.

In essence, cultivating or treating the Ghost Eyes point brings about clarity much like when dark clouds dissipate on a stormy day, allowing the sun to shine through to reveal what truly lies in front of you.

Liberating yourself from Ghost Eyes means you can genuinely engage in your current life experiences without being tainted by these hooks from the past.

Examine the life stories that might be limiting your freedom to live the way you want to be living. How do past events continue to impact your present-day existence?

Spend some time observing your life and how you might hold yourself back for fear of reliving negative experiences from the past, which is a natural post-traumatic stress response.

As you recognize the ways in which you are vigilantly protecting yourself, ask yourself what life could be like outside the fortress of protection you've built. Imagine shedding your armor. Would being unprotected feel too vulnerable? The lesson here is that the ultimate protection is connecting with the profound strength within yourself, eliminating the need for constant defense. Even if you can't let go of protection entirely, see if you can sense the freedom that living without constant vigilance would bring.

Clearing Ghost Eyes allows you to immerse yourself in the present moment, embracing life fully with an internal calm. You can allow events to unfold without that looming sense of dread and the need to be vigilantly scanning for potential dangers at all times.

Ghost Eyes Meditation

The purpose of this meditation is to identify any potential Ghosts or hooks that are functioning as lenses that obscure your vision and distort your perception of the world. These lenses reinforce the doubts associated with these Ghosts that obscure your authentic self and hinder your ability to see the world clearly. The goal of this meditation is to help you clear these obstructions, allowing you to see your life with clarity and without the interference of doubt.

You can begin by finding a quiet space and having your journal or notebook next to you for recording your reflections after the meditation. Then follow the *Relax Your Body and Clear Your Mind Meditation* on page 54 of this book. You can listen to the free guided version at the Alchemy Learning Center (AlchemyLearningCenter.com).

Once you are relaxed, take a few moments to clear your mind of any random thoughts that arise. Now you are ready to start the Ghost Eyes meditation.

Take a moment and think about one of your biggest doubts in life and which of the Nine Palaces it is related to. For example, is it a doubt concerning your career, your relationship, your health, or your abundance? Or is it something else?

What perspective do you have about these issues? Are you only noticing things in your life that confirm your doubts about the subject?

When Ghost Eyes are your lens to the world, the evidence supporting your doubts begins to become a story. This story becomes the basis of how you validate and protect the ghost's reality.

What story do you constantly tell yourself that is building a rigid, immovable fortress in support of that story?

Are there instances when your habitual viewpoint is overlooking aspects that support your truth? In the Health Palace, do your eyes only see signs of ill health? Are they not seeing the parts of you that are healthy? Identify the ways in which you are healthy. Even if the only spot on your body that feels healthy is your little toe, you can direct your attention there and affirm its good health.

In the Relationship Palace, do your eyes only see the ways you struggle with love and connection? What evidence is there that some of your relationships are working well in your life?

In your Career Palace, what aspects of your career are actually in alignment with your truth?

What do you have in your Wealth Palace, including things that aren't monetary, that indicate how much abundance you have in your life?

If you can't think of any evidence that supports your authentic truth, just think of the opposite of your doubts. Focus on what it would feel like if the exact opposite of your doubts were suddenly true. Think of a statement that would affirm that new feeling of truth.

Take a few minutes and really feel into what experiences support the real truth, discernible with that deep inherent knowing ability you were born with. *Your truth.*

When you are ready, you can open your eyes.

Make two columns in your journal—one for the doubts and one for the truth.

Now write down the evidence that supports the doubts in one column and the evidence that supports the truth in the other column.

For example, for the Health Palace, write down the evidence that created the feeling of ill health inside you. In the truth column write all the evidence and arguments that support your true health. This can be tricky if you feel like there is no evidence to support your truth. If that's the case, just think about what is the opposite of the doubts, and write that in the truth column as something you can affirm and manifest in the future.

You can listen to a guided version of this meditation at the Alchemy Learning Center (AlchemyLearningCenter.com).

Case Study: Lost and Found

When one of our clients had been college-age, long before she first came to see us, her parents had forced her to give up her baby for adoption. Over the years, she had carried a great deal of pain because of this loss. At some point, many years later, her son found her. But instead of letting go of the pain after their reconciliation, the story of the pain continued or may have even worsened. Now the son had become a constant reminder of the trauma of the past. Every time she saw him, she wanted to rejoice, but all she could remember was the years of pain and anguish the adoption had caused.

The initial part of the Ghost Point treatment seemingly reopened the wound that had already been reopened by the reconciliation as she recounted the events leading up to the birth. However, when we got to the Ghost Eyes point, she suddenly remembered how terrified she'd been to raise a child at such a young age. Suddenly, this thought opened up a sense of forgiveness for her parents and for her younger self. This point helped her to release the pain of the events that had led up to the adoption and her part in it. She began to see other viewpoints and was finally able to take steps to develop a deep connection with her grown son. It was as if she could finally see her son for who he truly was, and she could rejoice in his presence in her life, instead of seeing him as a symbol of her life-long pain.

The Second Trinity of Ghost Points – Your Inner World

The next three points show how once a "ghost" has hooked into a person, it begins to affect a person's internal world and change their true nature. The ghost begins to try to exhaust the person's yang energy so it can take over. Therefore, much of this second trinity is about tonifying the yang, to restore it.

At this depth, the "ghost" is starting to affect the person's Heart and the physical Kidney *Jing*/Essences. This relates to the concept of Heart/Kidney communication in Chinese Medicine, or Fire/Water communication.

As the "ghost" works its way in deeper, it now begins to control a person's relationships with others and to take over their life's direction by creating detours that the "ghost" wants to experience.

And then it gets in at a much deeper level, affecting subconscious or unconscious beliefs. As a result, this trinity of points is related to a variety of symptoms and conditions often resulting from previous trauma such as inflexibility, feeling entrenched in life, a lack of movement (remaining sedentary), being unable to make decisions, and appearing directionless. There may be symptoms such as engaging in self-harm behaviors like cutting or hitting, displaying ADHD-like issues, alternating between laughing and crying, and any number of other behavioral problems that are disruptive to everyday life.

The points in this trinity attempt to summon up the true yang qi of the person in order to push the "ghost" back out.

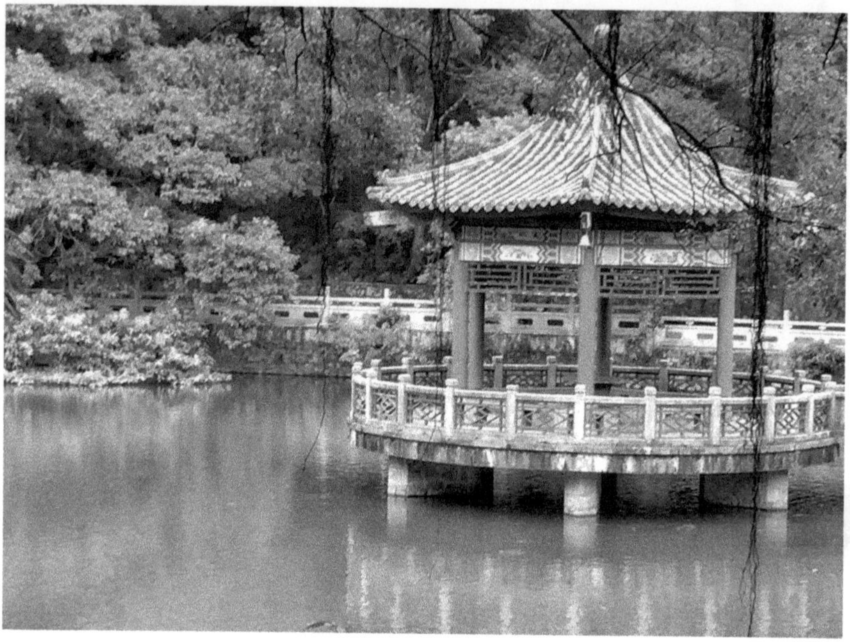

At the base of LuoFu Shan (Ge Hong's mountain), Huizhou, China

4 Ghost Heart – Gui Xin, Pericardium 7

Once the way you see the world has changed and the "ghost" has created its fortress within you, it now attempts to lock you out of your own heart. The "ghost" has infiltrated your heart and your emotional landscape, influencing how you *feel* about the world. Because your spirit lives in your heart, this means the "ghost" is now taking control of your spirit's home as well.

This shift might affect your feelings about your relationships with your loved ones, friends, co-workers, and close neighbors—especially how you communicate with them. Trust, once freely given, may now become much more difficult to achieve. Emotional manifestations such as suspicion, heartache, and defensiveness might surface in ways you've never experienced before.

Doubt has woven its way into every aspect of your existence. Everything and everyone is now subject to scrutiny, prompting a need to shield your heart—the very essence of your being—from a world that no longer feels safe. In the need for this defensive posture against the world, your sense of innocence has been lost, and the journey to recover it is blocked.

While the Ghost Points work with a concept of a progression or worsening of symptoms, when you experience heartbreak, it can cause the ghost to directly affect the heart, making the Ghost Heart the key point in this scenario.

When it comes to heartbreak, there's a whole range of different kinds of heart pain to think about. There's the classic cheating breakup, the gut-wrenching end of your first love, the devastating fallout with your best friend, the sad but somewhat mutual split, the one that got away and left you feeling empty inside, the painful death of a loved one, or the heartbreak of saying goodbye to a beloved pet.

And in today's world, there are some newer kinds of heartbreak that hit just as hard, like the crushing disappointment of realizing you've been scammed or catfished, and the love you felt turns out to be a total sham from the start, or the soul-crushing moment when someone you're crazy about ghosts you, vanishing from your life without a trace either online or offline. Then there's the sting of a hot hookup followed by a fade into nothingness, the heartbreak of meeting your instant soulmate—someone you're sure is "the one," only to have it fizzle out weeks later, or even the bitterness of a revenge breakup where love and anger become a tangled mess.

All of these and more can be addressed with Ghost Heart because in all these cases, your heart needs to heal and recover its ability to love again. Alternatively, you can use the point adjacent to Pericardium 7, which is Lung 9, a Metal point. Lung 9 is also called Ghost Heart. It works similarly to encourage the heart's ability to love again and might be good to add for a Metal Element person.

Indications

The Heart is the House of the Spirit, and at this point in the progression, the ghost has access to the Heart, thereby blocking the spirit from inhabiting its own home.

Eyes: The spirit in the Heart animates a person, enabling them to have light emanating from their eyes. When the "ghost" enters the eyes, the person may seem to lack expression and the brightness of the eyes may be dimmed.

Stuffy chest: The ghost may be blocking the chest, causing labored breathing or even what we call chest oppression, which can feel like a concrete block sitting on the chest.

Phlegm misting the Heart: In Chinese Medicine, phlegm in the body can begin to affect the Heart, causing mental illness. This is called "phlegm misting the Heart." This may mean that the person is no longer in control, which may look different for each person. Some common symptoms are: crying or weeping uncontrollably, laughing for no reason, or being irritable, hysterical, hostile, angry, or pathologically joyful. Many times these symptoms present as a bipolar-like pattern of alternating highs (mania) and lows (depression).

Irregular appetite: When the Heart is not free, the "ghost" begins to affect the appetite, either through loss of appetite and possibly not eating, or intense cravings and desires that can result in overeating. This can also translate into intense cravings and desires for non-food items, like binging screen time, excessive shopping, excessive drinking, or drug use.

Fear: When the "ghost" takes over a person's heart, the feeling of losing control can result in a generalized fear of everything. The person may even understand that the fear is irrational but not be able to release it.

Isolation: The person may begin to feel more isolated and want to be left alone, choosing not to do as much and preferring darkness and a generally more yin state.

Voice: The person's voice may be affected by the ghost in the Heart. It may sound more somber or stoic, more monotone or robotic, or like a little child's voice.

Treating Ghost Heart

Treating the Ghost Heart point liberates you from the shackles of heart pain, providing the opportunity to reopen your heart to the outer world. By letting go of a posture of defensiveness, you can begin to mend the fractures that have hindered your relationships, facilitating a return to a state where your heart can once again communicate freely.

This point harmonizes the stomach, unbinds the chest, calms the *Shen*/Spirit, and establishes the communication between the Heart and the Kidneys. It also addresses the tension between a person's materialistic and spiritual desires. For example, sometimes a heart's desire goes into the Kidneys, which are the seat of your constitution, and the desire morphs into an insatiable addiction. In this case, the Ghost Heart point will reconnect the Heart and Kidneys, while opening up the the upper and lower orifices to release whatever is contaminating the *Jing*/Essences.

Needling: 5 fen (.05 cun)

Energetic Approach: Use a vibrating light pressure on the point while focusing on the person's heart.

Moxibustion: When a person's spirit has lost its light, you can add moxibustion to bring light back to this excessive yin state. Direct moxibustion is preferred or you can use a moxa stick over the point. If the person is more manic and agitated, full of excess energy, or with wiry pulses, you do not need to add the moxibustion.

Ghost Heart Self-Cultivation

To cultivate this point, you can begin to examine what makes you feel defensive in life. What situations bring out your defensive postures? Is this a frequent occurrence or relatively rare? Is your heart protector always on guard, not allowing anyone in?

What are the ways you can begin to feel safe enough to reopen your heart to the outer world? Can you begin to mend your heart and return to a state where your heart can once again communicate freely?

Ghost Heart Meditation

The purpose of this meditation is to determine if the Ghosts from your past are causing your Heart Protector to work overtime in your relationships, overly protecting you and disconnecting you from your authentic self. In Chinese Medicine, we say the Heart must be connected to the Kidneys in order for you to be fully embodied and in alignment with yourself. When the Heart and Kidneys are disconnected, it feels like you're cut off from yourself or inaccessible to yourself. The goal of this meditation is to help you reconnect with your true qi and your Heart, enabling it to be open and free once again.

Begin by finding a quiet space and having your journal or notebook next to you for recording your reflections after the meditation. Then follow the *Relax Your Body and Clear Your Mind Meditation* on page 54 of this book. You can listen to this guided meditation at the Alchemy Learning Center (AlchemyLearningCenter.com).

Once you are relaxed, take a few moments to clear your mind of any thoughts that arise. Now you are ready to start the Ghost Heart meditation.

Take a moment and gently bring your attention to your heart. Focus your energy into your heart, the physical heart in your chest. Imagine your spirit that lives in the empty space inside your heart where the blood flows through. Let your awareness sit in your heart for a few minutes.

If you feel any agitation, just allow your heart to relax and let go. Let go of all the "to-do's" and desires you're holding onto. Simply be present with your heart.

Begin generating light in the darkness of the space inside your heart. It's a warm, reassuring light, and it begins to grow as you focus on it.

Now imagine that your heart has a membrane that protects the outside of it. This membrane is trying to protect you, but right now, you don't need protection. You are in a safe space.

As you occupy the space inside your heart where this warm light is glowing, imagine that you open that membrane up so that you can let the light inside you begin to emanate and shine out from you.

It may feel like a very small amount of light at first. Continue to open your heart and allow that light to grow and magnify outward.

Think about your interactions with people in your everyday life, especially those who feel safest to you—your family members or friends who genuinely love and care for you. How does your heart respond when you engage with them? Does it feel safe to express your authentic self and shine your inner light in their presence?

Even within these relationships, you might hesitate to open your heart for fear of being vulnerable. Take a few moments to assess your existing relationships and see if your heart feels free to be open and authentic in the presence of any or all of them.

Now, think about areas of your current life where you might not feel safe to be open and authentic with someone. What causes your Heart Protector to need to close your heart and protect you? Why does being vulnerable feel scary or unwise with certain people?

Ask yourself what happened in your past that makes you feel afraid or nervous to be vulnerable and open with these types of people.

Take a few minutes to reflect on any challenges you're facing in your relationships right now. Consider what past experiences might be influencing these current issues. Then bring into your mind any past or present relationships in which you have felt safe or imagine what it would be like to feel that way.

When you are ready, open your eyes.

In your journal, write down a list of the past issues that may have changed the way you now interact with people in your current life. How have you carried them with you? Could you consider shifting these perspectives? You can listen to this guided meditation at the Alchemy Learning Center (AlchemyLearningCenter.com).

5 Ghost Road – Gui Lu, Bladder 62

The Ghost Road point shows how a person, once hooked by a "ghost," no longer walks their true path in life. You may even start taking on a different appearance because you've begun taking on the form of the ghost.

One principle in Chinese Medicine is that every person has a destiny to fulfill in life, or what the Daoists call a curriculum. This is a lesson plan for fulfilling your individual purpose, which is the reason you have come into this incarnation.

It could be career-related, or you might have come in wanting to experience some particular aspect of life, perhaps by having a grand adventure. Perhaps you want to have a specific kind of relationship or have children.

Once a "ghost" has hooked into you, it now has control over your feet and the direction you will walk. This situation is what we call a blocked Will—when you have lost the Will to fulfill your own curriculum. When the Will is blocked, you can't stand up to the world to affirm your true self. You can't even stand up to yourself.

You may end up totally giving up on your dream, either because you don't think it's achievable, or because you simply become convinced that you no longer want to fulfill any of it.

Often a blocked Will can begin with an overbearing parent or partner who constantly tells you what to do. Over time, you stop being able to decide what you want to do anymore.

Perhaps out of fear or a sense of sacrifice, you may have taken a giant detour off your life's true path. Or even worse, you may have lost all your energy and desire to do anything at all! You may simply be frozen in fear. When you're frozen, you believe that staying still will prevent the bad outcome you've been trying to avoid. You might believe that your authentic road is now unsafe, so you choose instead to take a "safe" road instead, or you simply go somewhere to hide out and stay still so as to ensure that nothing bad can happen.

Indications

The signs and symptoms of the Ghost Road point indicate that the person no longer has enough yang to rid themselves of the "ghost."

Now the "ghost" has control of the person's feet and where they're walking in life. The person is no longer in charge of their motility (Bladder channel or *Qiao Mai*/Motility vessels). An example might be someone in recovery who has sworn not to go to the liquor store to buy alcohol and yet somehow, the car ends up in the liquor store parking lot. In other words, the person goes places they don't want to go because the ghost wants to revisit places from their previous lifetime. Or the ghost might also want to direct the person to go to places where ghosts typically hang out, like bars or hospitals, where people are unhappy or have recently died.

Sleep: The Bladder channel is connected to the eyes. When the Water Element in you doesn't feel safe, you may often feel the need to be vigilant. This may cause the person's eyes to stay open at night, resulting in insomnia, due to the need to be aware of the surroundings at all times.

Tension: As a person's ability to move (motility) becomes more compromised, the lateral/outside of the body can become very tense, while the medial/inside side can become flaccid/soft.

Restlessness: The person has difficulty settling down and may be pacing the room, especially at night. The person may be exhibiting more compulsive or uncontrollable behaviors.

Sensitive: The person may be easily startled, sensitive to light and sound, or simply be overwhelmed by too much activity in the environment.

Shutting down: The blood in the body is no longer flowing properly, so the person isn't interacting with the world as much. The qi of the body has become inert, causing a state known as qi stasis. This results in what we call "heat in the blood," which can cause more reactivity to circumstances in the world, resulting in mania or obsessive activity and not wanting to slow down. Other symptoms may include rebelliousness, aggression, or a tendency to want to fight or even be violent. Heat in the blood can stir up wind, causing seizures, convulsions, epilepsy, or loss of consciousness.

Broken blood vessels: These can appear on the jaw or around the Bladder 62 point under the outer ankle.

Eyes: There may be unusual eye symptoms, such as any misalignment, asymmetry, or other deviation of the eyes because the *Yin Qiao Mai* vessel goes to Bladder 1 at the inner canthus of the eye

Other symptoms: These may include general dizziness or vertigo, tremors, palpitations, Bell's palsy, paralysis, or projectile vomiting.

Treating Ghost Road

Treating the Ghost Road point thaws the frozen sensation of being stuck and gets the person's feet moving forward again along their road. It orients them onto the intended path they were meant to be walking, before they veered off course. It accomplishes this by reestablishing the will, which is the person's driving force behind fulfilling their purpose. Once they reconnect with that higher purpose, walking their authentic road becomes much easier.

Pericardium 7 is a Fire point that leads to Bladder 62, which is a Water point. So, in essence, the treatment is bringing the Fire to the Water. The movement from Pericardium 7 (Ghost Heart) to Bladder 62 (Ghost Road) connects the Heart and Kidney, enabling the "Heart to speak," meaning they can communicate what they really want and need to say out loud in the treatment. Sometimes they are able to tell stories they've never told anyone before, and just the speaking of their truth is a tremendous healing. This in turn allows them to better express their true selves out in the world.

This point also extinguishes or releases wind, which brings more ease into the body and into life, by relaxing and soothing tight muscles, especially those in the chest and throat, which may also be hampering the release of the emotions and attached stories through storytelling.

This point also invigorates the blood, which can then help release the *Shen*, which may be trapped in the person's heart. Once the Shen is no longer caged, it can be calmed and soothed.

Adding moxibustion here will also help to tonify the yang energy, because Bladder is a yang channel.

Because the Bladder clears the brain of contaminants and is the outlet for the Kidneys, this point helps to clear any contaminated water in the brain, which can be seen as the cause of some types of mental illness. It opens the upper portals (especially the eyes at Bladder 1) to release pathogens, and it can simultaneously encourage fluids to move downward to be released through opening the lower portals (especially through urination). It's a good idea to check if a person needs to use the restroom after this point is finished. One client claimed she had never urinated as much in her entire life as she did after this point.

Needling: 3-5 fen (.03-.05 cun) The Fire needle technique can add more Fire to the Water to help bring contaminants out. The exact approach that Sun SiMiao used for the Fire needle technique is debated. Some possibilities are:

1. Heat up the needle and then insert it the appropriate fen depth 3–7 times.

2. Either use acu-moxibustion (moxa on top of the needle) or do 7 cones of direct moxibustion on the point, followed by needling.

3. Blow warm air (human breath) on the needle after insertion.

4. Use the Fire-Burning Mountain technique to create the heat through moving the needle (these are called flashes), rather than using actual fire. To do this:

    a. Insert the needle one-third of the depth (representing Heaven) and lift and thrust it back in at this depth 7 times.

    b. Then insert the needle two-thirds of the depth (representing Humanity) and lift and thrust it again 7 times here.

    c. Then insert the needle the full depth (representing Earth) and lift and thrust 7 times.

    d. Needle all three levels 7 times each, equaling a total of 21 times. This technique was traditionally used to treat cold deficiency, which is often present with a Will Block.

Energetic Approach: To simulate these possible needle actions with acupressure, you can take a number of approaches.

1. Vibrate your finger on the point while holding a moxa stick next to your finger and the point to warm both your finger, acting as the needle, and the point. Use a more vigorous vibrating technique than with other Ghost Points to stimulate and warm the point, simulating the Fire Needle technique.

2. Do the above technique as a Fire-Mountain technique by using three levels of pressure (Heaven, Humanity, and Earth) for a total of 21 times with a lifting and thrusting motion. You can alternate lighter pressure for the lifting out and deeper pressure for the thrust going inward. Because we do Bladder 62 for a much longer period of time than 21 flashes would take, you should continue to stimulate the point vigorously after the flashes are done, until the point is completed.

3. Do 7 direct moxa cones followed by vibrating the point with your finger.

Moxibustion: While the point requires more stimulation or heat than the earlier Ghost Points, moxibustion is not always necessary. Adjust the use of moxa according to the person's signs and symptoms by using tongue and pulse diagnosis. We often start the point without moxibustion and see if it feels inert or unresponsive and needs extra stimulation, either through more vigorous vibration or with moxibustion.

Ghost Road Self-Cultivation

Cultivating Ghost Road begins with examining how you move through the world and whether you're walking your true road. Have you been walking the path through life that you've wanted to walk? Or do you feel like you've been on a detour at times?

Sometimes this means you have to stand up for yourself because you've allowed certain patterns to take control over you. For example, the compulsiveness of addictions to food, alcohol, or over-spending. Do you have control over your own behavior?

It's also important to examine whether fear has played a big part in directing your path, perhaps leading you away from your authentic destiny path. This may mean that you have a Will Block that prevents you from walking your true road in life. If that's the case, then this point will dig into the deepest levels of fear that are obstructing your will to move forward and fulfill your life's purpose. In some cases, a Will Block even obstructs your sense of purpose and brings about a state of confusion about your destiny in general. However, once the fear is released, you'll be able to reconnect with your higher purpose and walk your true road once again.

Ghost Road Meditation

The purpose of this meditation is to explore and discover whether you are walking on your authentic life path—the road that aligns with your essential being's aspirations. What is your true destiny?

This meditation is designed to help you to discern whether past experiences are derailing you onto detours or blocking you from your true destiny. What are the potential "ghosts" that may be diverting you from your genuine path? While your destination might appear nebulous or distant, your next steps should feel clear when you're walking your true road.

You can begin by finding a quiet space and having your journal or notebook next to you for recording your reflections after the meditation. Then follow the *Relax Your Body and Open Your Doors Meditation* on page 54 of this book. You can listen to the recorded meditation at the Alchemy Learning Center (AlchemyLearning center.com).

Once you are relaxed, take a few moments to clear your mind of any thoughts that arise. Now you are ready to start the Ghost Road meditation.

Begin the meditation by taking a moment to settle into your heart, the tangible heart in your chest. Now direct your attention gently there. Envision your spirit residing in the empty space within your heart where the blood circulates. Allow your awareness to rest within your heart for a few moments.

Reflect on your life's journey—the authentic road leading to your destiny. Consider where you've come from along your road. Have there been instances in the past that hampered your ability to stay on course, possibly leading you away from your truest destiny?

What specific events or thoughts from your past have caused deviations in your life's trajectory? What might even be presently steering you off course? Select a specific event or recurring story that strongly feels like the most significant interference with your current journey.

Imagine that you are flying in a plane high above and can see the roads, the paths, and even the little side trails of your life below. Where do you think you would like to be going in the future? Ask yourself, "What is the road that feels most in alignment with my most authentic path—my Dao?"

The answer doesn't have to be very specific or well-defined. If you're going to the ocean, you don't have to know the specific beach you're going to... yet. You just have to know that you're headed to the ocean. This is the ambition of your Water Element. It's not a goal. It's your destiny—your desired destination.

When you're ready you can open your eyes and try to recall some of what you discovered in this meditation. Take a moment and write down some thoughts about your discoveries in your journal.

Some questions to consider are: What beliefs do you have about life that are based on the interference you identified? How has holding those beliefs changed your past trajectory, or the way you walk through life currently? What would you change today if you could?

You can listen to this guided meditation at the Alchemy Learning Center (AlchemyLearningCenter.com).

6 Ghost Pillow – Gui Zhen, Du 16

Ghost Pillow delves into the impact of the "ghost" on your sleep and your unconscious beliefs. The ghost has now entrenched itself deeply, altering the very nature of your unconsciousness. It's as if you're actually now sharing your sleep time with the ghost.

A pillow symbolizes comfort when you sleep, and part of that comfort creates a sense of safety that allows you to shut down your senses to the outside world. But when the "ghost" reaches the level of your unconscious, it begins affecting your ability to sleep deeply. Now, not only the outer world but also the inner world may feel unsafe, and it becomes difficult to let go into a sound sleep. This point is normally named Warehouse of Wind, indicating much agitation, as if the wind is blowing at night and you're trying to sleep in the middle of a storm. This point helps to regulate the wind.

You might feel as if you always have to keep one ear listening for danger in the night. It's as if someone yanked the pillow out from under your head and sleeping is no longer comforting. When the "ghost" gets in at this level, you might wake up feeling just as tired as when you went to bed.

You may not even be aware of the unconscious beliefs affecting you, such as thinking there are potential threats all around. This level of vigilance can certainly interrupt your ability to sleep deeply.

As the treatment progresses towards the Third Trinity, we now see that the person's yin is also being consumed with many more serious symptoms.

Indications

The "ghost" now has access to the deep unconscious, which means that the symptoms are becoming much more all-encompassing.

Fear: The person generally may be experiencing more fear and anxiety with a generalized lack of feeling safe, for no reason. This level of discomfort may result in being unwilling or unable to adapt to situations. The person may be very sensitive to what people are saying as well, even thinking people are being intentionally mean when they aren't.

Sleep: The person is now dreaming the ghost's dreams, which may seem like nightmares. Symptoms may include insomnia, sleep apnea, or dreams that make no sense to the person but might make sense to the ghost.

Mouth: This point and the next point address symptoms related to the mouth and jaw, such as TMJ, grinding teeth, trigeminal neuralgia, deviation of the mouth (such as with Bell's palsy), tooth decay, loss of sense of smell or voice, or a strange continuous talking without stopping (called "snake tongue" in Chinese Medicine).

Balance: As the "ghost" takes over the gait of the person and becomes in charge of the body's movement, the person may experience difficulty walking, dizziness, a feeling of being uncoordinated, or even gait disorders (loss of the person's normal gait).

Suicidal: The person may feel completely disengaged with the world and even come to the point of feeling like death is the best way to change the situation (called Death Wind).

Other symptoms: The person may experience any number of additional symptoms in extreme cases, such as paralysis, memory loss, holding onto to emotional issues, having a complete lack of compassion, having no awareness of others, or being unable to comply with social norms (even taking off their clothes and running around naked). The person may even behave like a totally different person or have violent episodes.

Treating Ghost Pillow

Treating the Ghost Pillow point accesses the deepest level of a person's unconscious and shakes up the unconscious beliefs. Points located on the head are considered to be more advanced than arm and leg points for beginner practitioners. So the progression itself is indicating that the "ghost" has advanced considerably.

Often while this point is being treated, the person drops into a deep meditative state. While many Ghost Points work better if the person talks (we always say the Heart needs to speak), this point in particular seems to require the person to take a verbal pause and go into a deep state of quiet. From there, if something bubbles up from the unconscious and needs to be spoken, then it's helpful to speak at that point.

For this reason it can be difficult to ascertain the immediate effect of this point. However, for some people it can be extremely profound. They may go into an almost trance-like state and when they return from that state, they often report profound sensations and visions that contribute to a feeling of peace.

Ghost Pillow (Du 16) extinguishes wind and evokes sweating and purging outward.

Needling: 10 fen (1 cun)[18] — You can optionally add the Fire needle technique without moxibustion, which is contraindicated for this point.

Energetic Approach: With the person lying supine (face up), cup the head with one hand while stimulating the point with your other hand's forefinger or middle finger.

---

[18] It is unclear in the original Chinese version whether the point is located 1 cun above the hairline or the needling depth is 1 cun.

Ghost Pillow Cultivation

Points on the head represent heaven and opening up to spirituality.

Cultivating this point helps you access your deepest unconscious level and potentially release some unconscious beliefs or memories that may be holding you back.

It's important when using this point on yourself to go slow and be gentle with yourself. You might not know what's buried inside you, and you need to act as your own practitioner, willing to listen to the stories that surface, even if they are disturbing. Approach this process without judgment and without dismissing anything that feels threatening to your current way of life or seems trivial. Honor whatever comes up with the same kindness that you would readily offer to another person.

Ghost Pillow Meditation

This meditation is designed to eliminate any limiting or inauthentic beliefs that may have taken root in your unconscious mind. For an optimal experience, we recommend lying down if possible and applying gentle vibrating pressure at the point (Du 16) at the center of the base of your occiput with your forefinger or middle finger, creating a subtle, slow vibration.

You can begin by finding a quiet space and having your journal or notebook next to you for recording your reflections after the meditation. Then follow the *Relax Your Body and Clear Your Mind Meditation* on page 54 of this book. You can listen to the guided meditation in the Alchemy Learning Center (AlchemyLearningCenter.Com).

Once you are relaxed, take a few moments to clear your mind of any thoughts that may arise. Now you are ready to start the Ghost Pillow meditation.

Relax your body and your mind while practicing deep, rhythmic breathing. Begin to apply gentle vibrating pressure at the center of the base of your occiput with your forefinger or middle finger. The idea is to create a slow and subtle vibration at the base of your skull.

As you continue vibrating your finger, allow yourself to begin to gradually delve into your subconscious mind. Reaching this level can feel like the sensation of drifting off to sleep, free of thoughts.

Allow yourself to fully relax your mind and descend even deeper from your subconscious mind down into your unconscious mind, while breathing more and more peacefully. After a few minutes, see if you can encourage yourself to go deeper still, reaching a state where you cannot consciously direct your thoughts, although they may surface spontaneously.

Spend the next few minutes in this state, observing any and all thoughts that may emerge.

When you're ready, you can slowly come back up to the subconscious mind level, by slowly bringing your breath back to its normal breathing pattern.

Now, come all the way back to your conscious mind and slowly open your eyes. Return to the world around you.

Take note of any thoughts that arose during this journey. Write them down as a reflection of your experience.

You can listen to this guided meditation at the Alchemy Learning Center (AlchemyLearningCenter.com).

Summary of First and Second Trinities

The progression of these initial six points delineates how a person gets infiltrated by a "ghost," often stemming from from past trauma and negative experiences. This ghost might be something that got into the system from the outside, like an entity or a parasite, or it could be something internally generated, such as chronic stress, emotional states or unconscious beliefs that do not serve the person. Once this ghost gets into the system, it gradually becomes more and more entrenched in the body/mind/spirit and "hooks into" the person, becoming very difficult to release. Once hooked in, it buries itself deeper into the psyche, affecting behaviors, relationships, self-esteem, and unconscious beliefs.

From the perspective of our spiritual growth, these points can provide insights into pathways for reclaiming our authentic selves. These points guide us in understanding the steps required to find truer states of authenticity.

The Third Trinity of Ghost Points – Heart Pains

The next three Ghost Points represent the way the "ghost" buries itself into the very deepest part of a person, affecting the ability to sleep to an even stronger degree, as well as the ability to speak about oneself in the world. Finally, the "ghost" gains access to the inner heart.

The initial six points within the Thirteen Ghost Points protocol may effectively address mild blockages. However, for individuals who have endured severe trauma or abuse, a comprehensive approach encompassing the entire protocol is often necessary for significant healing.

As the "ghost" embeds itself even deeper into the system, the yin parts of the physical body, such as the fluids and the essences, may endure more harm. This may result in the person isolating more from the world and not wanting people in their lives, increasing levels of mental illness, self-harming, perhaps not speaking or eating, or becoming a danger to society. The third trinity attempts to repair the damaged Yin.

Case Study: Hand-wringing

One elderly, single man came to us with a history of some mild signs of anxiety. It had progressed slowly but then took a sudden turn for the worse. He began wringing his hands, was unable to sleep, and was sure he was dying, even though there was no apparent reason. His biggest issue was that the anxiety was too great for him to travel, which made it impossible for him to see his grandchildren.

His anxiety was so extreme that he repeatedly called an ambulance for help. However, the doctors found nothing wrong physically, although he did suffer from constipation. They prescribed medications for the constipation and the anxiety, but he had been too afraid to take either of them.

During the Ghost Points treatment, he continued to fret and wring his hands in the beginning, but then, during the

Third Trinity, it was as if the light had returned to his eyes. He started talking about things he used to like to do and the people in his life he used to engage with. He stopped fretting about his situation. And by the last point, he was in a completely calm state.

When he came in for his follow-up, he was excited and was no longer wringing his hands. He felt like himself again. He was looking forward to getting back to a full life, including traveling and seeing his grandchildren. Over the next year, that's exactly what he did. He began to rebuild his life and started adventuring out into the world again, and even began to date someone.

7 Ghost Bed – Gui Chuang, Stomach 6

The next two points are in the mouth area because the "ghost" is trying to take over the person's communication in order to express itself. In order to do this, it begins to consume the yin of the body. It also takes over the person's inner voice that they use to talk to themself.

As a result, that voice becomes overwhelmed by obsessive thinking and worry, which can be sourced in past trauma and negative experiences. This worry shows up at bedtime, often resulting in insomnia due to the obsessive thinking. At this point, the person is no longer able to sort out what is good or bad for them in the world.

This means the body's natural detoxification process isn't working, and this causes the negative emotions to be stored in the blood. In Chinese Medicine theory, too many negative emotions in the system can affect the blood in the system, turning it darker, even purple. This is called blood stasis.

So if that negative emotion is anger, and we are angry at a person or at the world, and won't let it go, that anger is going to go into our blood and turn the color of the blood from a bright healthy red to a darker red or even purple.

Indications

This point begins the second half of the treatment and indicates the damaging effects the "ghost" can now have on the body as the yin is being consumed. More obsessions emerge due to an underlying feeling that the person's health is slipping away.

While the corresponding symptoms can seem extreme, we believe that most people in today's world (even those without diagnosed mental health issues) have some amount of obsessive thinking that can be lessened by the use of this point.

Face: The damage to the yin of the body may contribute to tooth decay. The body tends to store toxins in the teeth that would otherwise result in illness if they were stored in other parts of the body. Other related symptoms may include: jaw clenching, TMJ, trigeminal neuralgia, teeth chattering, foaming at the mouth, difficulty chewing, dark rings around the eyes, and facial tics.

Obsessive thinking: It becomes more and more difficult for the person to let things go. This is symbolized by the point's location on the jaw, causing teeth grinding, like a cow chewing on its cud, over and over again. This works for a cow's digestion of food but not for a person's digestion of their thoughts. Mentally, the mind is repetitively chewing on its own thoughts. This results in a lack of compassion for others because the person can't stop fixating on their own problems, let alone be concerned about someone else's.

Sleep: Due to obsessive thinking, the person becomes unable to sleep. This may include a lot of tossing and turning in bed while constantly worrying about anything and everything.

Body: As the "ghost" begins to damage the body's yin essences, the person may begin to feel very cold. The person may also lose a lot of weight and look as if they're wasting away. Sometimes the belly is swollen with a drum-like distention, while the arms and legs appear skinny. At this point the person may have parasites or candida due to fermentation in the gut. There may be a loss of appetite, loss of muscle tone, a stiff spine, more phlegm in the system, projectile vomiting, and overall malnourishment.

Treating Ghost Bed

As we said the "ghost" is now consuming the body's yin. The goal of treating this point is to nourish, safeguard, and protect the yin, which is called *Bao Yin* in Chinese.

Traditionally this point was lanced to release the dark blood related to worry and obsessive thinking.

Treating this point can free a person of obsessive thinking in general and relieve whatever is causing them to "chew" on things over and over again.

When someone has deep intense emotions, bloodletting in general (especially on the *Luo* points) can help. But this point actually releases the underlying reasons for the dark blood. If someone is self-harming, for example by purposely cutting themselves, they are performing a form of bloodletting, which may be helping them release their trapped emotions. This release would be much better and more safely managed through acupuncture, but in both cases, bloodletting of any kind only releases a little bit of the painful emotions at a time. Ghost Bed (Stomach 6), on the other hand, attempts to release a deeper underlying level of pain, so the person won't have the inclination to cut anymore.

Needling: Sun SiMiao indicated that this area of the jaw should actually be lanced. You would begin by massaging the area around Stomach 6 to get the blood to release, then lance the point and gently squeeze the blood out. The color of the blood indicates the level of negative emotions stored in the blood. The darker the blood, the more negativity in the system.

Optionally, you can use the Fire needle technique, using a warm bleeding needle. This might mean heating up the needle before lancing or heating up the area (for example, with a moxa stick) and then lancing. In either case, massaging the area first is important because it activates the salivary glands to generate fluids. The person may feel as if they've eaten something tart, like a lemon.

Energetic Approach: One of the more advanced techniques you can do with the energetic needling approach is a "bleeding" technique. When not using a lance or needle, you're obviously not going to get any blood out. However, many years ago, Leta discovered this technique with a client who had a blood blister below her wrist along the Lung meridian. Acupuncturists would traditionally bleed the *Luo* point associated with that meridian (Lung 7) to release any dark stagnant blood in the channel. Leta decided to try "bleeding" the point energetically. She first made a psychic "cut," imagining that her finger was a lance, to energetically open the point. Then she began squeezing the negativity out of the point, imagining gray/black energy oozing out of the point. To her and her client's astonishment, the blister disappeared right before their eyes. This has become the method we now use and teach for the Ghost Bed Point.

To do the technique with your fingertip, psychically lance the point to make a tiny invisible outlet for the energy to come out. Then begin physically squeezing the skin to release the negative energy or qi out of the point, as if there were dark blood coming out. Instead of actual blood, you move the negative energy that the blood contains out through the outlet you created. You may even feel some tingling sensations or the client may feel them.

Sun SiMiao did not indicate the Stomach 6 point directly but a specific distance (5 or 8 fen) beneath the ear lobe, which is around the Stomach 6 point. For this reason, we massage the whole area around Stomach 6, from the cheekbone to the neck and from the mouth to the ear. Continue to palpate and massage the cheeks and jaw area, working towards the Stomach 6 points on both sides to release negative stress and qi. Optionally you can massage the inside of the mouth (with gloves if required). Continue to do this until the point feels resolved.

Optional Additional Technique: While not part of Sun SiMiao's Thirteen Ghost Point prescription, we like to sometimes follow up with a more tonifying approach for someone who is very depleted. You can either add moxibustion via a moxa stick, or simply a tonifying non-needle vibrating technique with your finger. The intention is to nourish the yin if the person does have symptoms of damaged yin.

Ghost Bed Cultivation

To cultivate this point in your life, examine your mind and the way it's talking to you about your life. Our minds can take over and tell us things that aren't actually true or authentic to ourselves. Take your time with this process. This may be the result of years of mental patterns that may take some time to unravel.

As you work through this point for personal growth, you begin to release the tension stored in your jaw or you may find you're clenching your jaw less. This is an indication that your efforts are working. For example, let's say you're trying to accomplish something in your life, but you used to feel like you were constantly being thwarted. As you work with this point, you may develop a sense of peace about the outcome, like a knowing that it's going to work out just fine.

Use the following meditation to help shift your perspective.

Ghost Bed Meditation

The goal of this meditation is to examine the things you're obsessively thinking about or worrying about and to give them over to the "Divine Concierge" to handle.

You can begin by finding a quiet space and having your journal or notebook next to you for recording your reflections after the meditation. Then follow the *Relax Your Body and Clear Your Mind Meditation* on page 54 of this book. You can listen to the guided meditation in the Alchemy Learning Center (AlchemyLearningCenter.com).

Once you are relaxed, take a few moments to clear your mind of any thoughts that arise. Now you are ready to start the Ghost Bed meditation.

Relax your mind deeply while practicing deep, rhythmic breathing. In this fully relaxed state, ask yourself what thoughts or worries you have that you keep returning to over and over. What thoughts particularly disturb your sleep because you can't put them to rest, even at night?

After you examine these thoughts, imagine they are all things that you can easily put in a backpack. Take all of these worries and obsessions and put them in your imaginary backpack right now.

Now imagine you're standing in a room that is all white. In the center of the room is a large table. The room belongs to the Divine Concierge who works for the Divine and is at your service to take care of anything you want or need.

Walk over to the table and put your backpack on it. Whatever you put into that backpack, the Divine Concierge will now take care of. Open the backpack and unpack all the unwanted things you placed in it. The Divine Concierge will handle everything for you. You just simply drop off your obsessions with no worries, assured that they will be taken care of in the perfect way. You can go on your merry way and have fun, without needing to think about them anymore.

Spend the next five minutes feeling what it would be like to walk out of that room knowing that the Universe is handling all these worrisome things for you. Imagine not obsessively thinking about them anymore. Feel how freeing this is. Feel the flow of the Universe. Feel the ease.

When you're ready you can open your eyes and return to the world around you.

Take note of any thoughts that arose during this journey. Write them down as a reflection on your experience.

You can listen to this guided meditation at the Alchemy Learning Center (AlchemyLearningCenter.com).

8 Ghost Market – Gui Shi, Ren 24

This point focuses on how you speak about yourself in the world. Does what you say come across well or turn people away? We are always needing to explain ourselves to others. Essentially, we are presenting ourselves, like a vendor at the market. So, are you speaking truly about yourself in a loving way, or do you tend to sometimes denigrate yourself?

Imagine that you are a vendor at a bustling Farmer's Market with crates of luscious apples to sell that you grew with love and care. If you go around telling everyone about the worms that are occasionally found in your apples, chances are you won't sell very many apples! Instead, as the apple seller, you would be accentuating the positives—their beautiful glossy skins, their juiciness, their sweetness—all the things that make these apples irresistible.

That doesn't mean you have to sweep the negatives under the rug. You're not trying to convince someone who might not like your apples to buy them anyway. Ghost Market represents the ability to be honest in a way that helps the right person to become aware of your gifts. Perhaps, with a playful wink, you can say to your customers, "These apples are the tastiest around. In fact, they're so good, even the worms can't resist a nibble now and then."

Ghost Market is about recognizing and valuing yourself and what you have to offer the world. It helps shift a negative outlook that may have originated from others' negativity or your own critical self-assessment. This negativity often manifests in statements like, "I'm flighty," "I'm not that smart," or "I'm not reliable." People frequently talk more about their perceived flaws than their strengths, a habit you'll notice in many of your clients as they speak about themselves.

Indications

While the signs and symptoms for this point may sound extreme, we believe that most people in today's world have difficulty speaking about themselves at all and rarely do so in a positive way. Almost everyone can find this point beneficial.

Dampness: The person's body at this point may be overcompensating for the loss of yin by being drawn to addictive foods that dampen the body, such as foods with added sweeteners, in order to bring back moisture/yin. Or the person may be taking higher doses of antidepressants, which suppress the yang qi in the body, causing the fluids to build up. This can result in swollen glands and an inability to digest well.

Dryness: It is also possible that the person's mouth may be very dry, and they may want to drink water all the time, as if there were no way to quench their thirst. The person may be attracted to drying foods (such as spicy, dehydrated, or air-fried food) as well as alcohol or caffeine. These drying foods can further dry up bodily fluids.

Heat: As the yin is depleted, the heat in the body may increase, causing dark urine or even nosebleeds.

Wasting: The person might feel as though their body is deteriorating or wasting away, a sign of damaged yin. In severe cases, they may have an emaciated appearance, especially if an actual entity (*Gui*/ghost) is involved. Alternatively, they might simply feel utterly exhausted. This condition can manifest as a general lack of appetite or, conversely, extreme hunger as the body attempts to restore its yin through eating. Additionally, the person might experience a loss of bodily control, such as what occurs after a stroke.

Mental state: The person's mental state may further deteriorate at this point, with signs of mania, hand-wringing, or even periods of rage. The classical symptom for this point would be running around naked in the streets.

Parasites: The person is more vulnerable to parasites due to the extreme hunger and resultant overeating, creating a vicious cycle where the parasites then need more food to consume.

Additionally, the teeth grinding symptom associated with Ghost Bed may increase the desire to chew in general, leading to cravings for crunchy foods.

Treating Ghost Market

Treating Ghost Market can help a person authentically find the words that represent them best, so that they can connect with the people out in the world that need their gifts.

To do this, a person first needs to appreciate what their strengths are. Finding the right words for one's strengths can be challenging for most people due to societal norms that require false humility in day-to-day conversation. Ren 24 is also called the Saliva or Sauce Receiver, meaning it's a receptacle for the verbal "sauce" that we're cooking up. In other words, it's about how we are going to speak about ourselves. Is it going to be a good sauce? Ghost Market helps people focus on just the right balance between highlighting the benefits of their gifts and what they can do for other people, without seeming to brag or overpromise something that they actually can't deliver.

Similar to Ghost Bed, this point nourishes, safeguards, and protects the yin also called *Bao Yin* in Chinese.

Needling: 2-3 fen (0.2-0.3 cun)

Energetic Approach: While facing the person, use your finger to lightly stimulate the point while conversing. You may need to prop your arm up with pillows.

Case Study: What a Year a Ghost Point Makes!

In our experience, Ren 24 is a point that can profoundly benefit clients without triggering overwhelming reactions. Although you may not be able to unlock its full potential without doing the preceding points in the protocol, the results of doing the single point can still be astonishing. Leta once did this point for a woman at an expo during a brief 20-minute treatment at her booth. A year later, the woman returned, recounting a life-transforming experience. She believed that the treatment had changed her entire life and she now had everything she wanted. She felt that the point had dissolved a barrier that had been hindering her progress in the past, and that now, without that barrier, she had been able to speak her truth and go after what she truly wanted—to move across the country, find her romantic partner, and have the career she'd always dreamed of. All that from one Ghost Point!

Ghost Market Cultivation

This point helps you to express yourself authentically and positively so that you can effectively communicate your message to those who could benefit from your gifts and talents.

To further cultivate this point, a good Ghost Market exercise is to craft your "elevator speech," or what you would say about yourself to a stranger during a brief elevator encounter.

This does not necessarily have to be about your career, although that is often how society encourages us to speak about ourselves with our most common opening question being, "What do you do for a living?" Instead, your elevator pitch can very well be about you as a person and how you conduct your personal life.

Think about what unique gifts you possess and how you contribute them to the world. How could you convey this information to others or even to yourself, without either denigrating or over-aggrandizing yourself?

Ghost Market Meditation

The purpose of this meditation is to find the best way to speak about yourself in the world so your gifts can be better received by those who need them.

You can begin by finding a quiet space and having your journal or notebook next to you for recording your reflections after the meditation. Then follow the *Relax Your Body and Clear Your Mind Meditation* on page 54 of this book. You can listen to the guided meditation in the Alchemy Learning Center (AlchemyLearningCenter.com).

Imagine yourself having a bunch of delicious apples you've grown with loving care. You invested a great deal of your time and energy tending them, watering them, fertilizing them, protecting them from birds and insects, and much more. These apples represent your unique gifts that you want to share with others. Now think about how you'd tell people about these special apples so the people who need them can find them.

Some people will love your apples and may even need your apples, and some may not. It's okay that not everyone is right for your apples and all that they offer! What's important is that you speak about them in a way that the people who might like them will take notice and consider buying them.

Ghost Market is located just below the mouth and is about speaking. Imagine how you would tell people about your apples? Would you talk about the quality of them? Would you talk about the taste? What are the features that you think people are going to appreciate the most?

Then what would you say about these attributes? Would you say that your apples are beautiful to look at but taste kind of mealy? Or would you proudly tell everyone that these are the best-tasting apples in the whole world and even better if you like a little texture.

Would you say, "My apples are great but there are a lot of worms in them?" Or would you say, "My apples are the best-tasting apples. In fact, even though you might find an occasional worm in them, it's only because the worms know which apples are the tastiest. So if you're a person who wants the tastiest apples, my apples are the ones for you."

The truth is, some people might prefer the flavor of your apples, and some people might prefer other apples. And that's okay.

Now think about your own special gifts to the world. If you met someone who could really benefit from what you offer, how would you describe it to them? You don't need to feel as if you are bragging or exaggerating or even trying to convince them. You only need to share what is true in a positive light that feels genuine and doesn't turn the person off. What can you say that will inspire them to take a look at what you offer?

Sometimes, it might feel hard to talk positively about yourself without feeling like you should add something negative. The negativity is the ghost taking over your mouth and saying, don't bother with these gifts, they're no good.

Take a few moments, while holding and vibrating the point Ren 24, located on the crease below your bottom lip, to imagine what you could say about your gifts. Allow the point to clear the negativity, so that you can feel the value of what you have to offer to the right recipients who will truly appreciate your gifts.

When you're ready you can open your eyes and return to the present world around you.

Take a moment to write down the positive statements that may have come to you during this journey. Write them down as a reflection on your experience. You can listen to this guided meditation at the Alchemy Learning Center (AlchemyLearningCenter.com).

9 Ghost Cave – Gui Ku, Pericardium 8

Ghost Cave is the point Pericardium 8, which is also called the Palace of Weariness or the Palace of Taxation. At this stage, the person is exhausted by all the effort they've put into trying to get life back to normal.

Ghost Cave is not about the people around you. It's more about your internal reality, which is different from the previous Pericardium point (Ghost Heart or Pericardium 7), which focuses on your relationships and how you communicate.

Think of Ghost Cave as the very heart of your heart—who you truly are in this incarnation of this lifetime. The Pericardium is the outer part of the heart—the walls that protect that cave we're talking about. The Pericardium's job is to decide when it's safe to open the heart and when it's not. When the Pericardium shuts down, the spirit can't flow freely.

Sometimes the past just weighs heavily on your heart. Those old memories dig their claws in and won't let go. We all have things in the past that sting to think about. And according to Chinese Medicine, when we hang onto all the hurts, it actually clogs up our blood flow.

In Chinese Medicine terms, this is what's called blood stagnation—when our heart's blood can't flow freely because of the accumulated emotions like grief and grudges clinging to our insides. We want to forgive, maybe even try to forget, but some wounds don't heal easily, especially when something truly awful happened, like the kind of abuse that shreds a person's soul. That kind of trauma doesn't let go easily.

The center of the heart (the Cave) is an empty space through which the blood flows. This space or Cave is your spirit's home, and ideally your spirit should move freely about inside it, without restriction.

When your blood flows through this hollow space, your spirit infuses it with life force, giving the blood its vibrant red color. The pumping mechanism of the heart circulates the spirit via the blood throughout your body, imbuing you with spirited energy. The spirit-infused blood imparts a sense of vitality and makes you feel truly alive.

Ghost Cave is treated when the "ghost" has taken up residence within your heart and become the sovereign ruler of your palace. To maintain a free and unfettered spirit, it's crucial to avoid becoming hooked by this "ghost." Once the "ghost" has gotten in this deep, you're likely to have a lot of heart pain that's not necessarily tied to external circumstances currently happening around you. It can feel like a heavy weight you have to carry.

Treating Ghost Cave clears out the accumulated debris that has collected in the heart and the arteries—strong and unrelenting memories of disappointments, guilt, and traumatic experiences that you just can't stop thinking about. These must be moved out so that the blood and the spirit can move freely again.

The truth is that while you can be injured physically and emotionally, the spirit can never be injured or harmed in any way. Your actual spirit always remains intact and unaffected. It can, however, be displaced but only when the home of the spirit, which is the heart, is hurt or damaged. In other words, the home of your spirit is the heart, and we experience heartbreak whenever we feel emotionally injured. Just as a physically blocked artery can prevent the proper circulation of the blood, the emotional pain that is stuck in your heart interferes with the heart's ability to circulate the spirit via the blood.

When we label someone as "mean-spirited" for causing us harm, it's because their actions feel like an assault on our spirit, and we feel hurt. Then the heart is no longer free the way it was before the hurt. When these heart pains accumulate in the "cave" of our hearts, they obstruct the free movement of the spirit.

If the spirit is inherently impervious to injury of any kind, then the only thing that can go wrong is that its free flow through the body can become obstructed. When it's blocked, it's not free to do what it's supposed to do. Then you might feel emotionally shut down or even inaccessible to yourself, which means the block is so big that now you can't even access your own inner sense of self. It's at this point that people will often say "I'm broken" or "I'm heartbroken." What that really means is that your spirit can't move freely around the body like it used to.

The questions to ask yourself are: Is your spirit free and making you feel alive and vital? And if not, is there some kind of roadblock? If so, what's blocking the free movement of your spirit?

Case Study: Evoking Anger

Treating Ghost Cave can elicit extreme reactions in some clients and even from the people around them. One client had suffered very painful childhood abuse throughout his childhood. When Leta used this point in his treatment, she was surprised to recognize that an overwhelming feeling of anger came over her. It was an interesting sensation, because there was no reason for her to feel angry with this client, and it made no sense to Leta. He wasn't doing or saying anything that would trigger a feeling of anger. However, the point was releasing something within the client that was oddly evoking an energetic feeling and reaction in Leta.

He reported later to Leta that after he left his appointment, his energy evoked anger in others who came into contact with him. In fact, everywhere he went, people responded angrily and yelled at him—the cashier at the grocery store, the gas station attendant, even his spouse reacted with rage when he arrived home. It was as if his inner turmoil was projecting outward and being mirrored back by the world around him.

The term for this is *resonance*, where internal energies manifest externally. In this case, it was almost as if the deep trauma encoded in his body from the abuse was emitting a painful frequency to the rest of the world, like fingernails on a blackboard.

When Ghost Cave releases these blocked energies, they can ripple out into the world around you. This is why this point requires more advanced training to utilize as a ghost point in a clinical setting. Once the pain, rage, or grief that was lodged in the heart is cleared, it opens up the ability for the heart to connect lovingly again with others.

Rewriting Your Autobiography Exercise

The Ghost Cave point connects to the deeper stories and narratives we carry that shape our view of self and world. Ghost Cave is located on the Pericardium meridian, and the Pericardium acts as a bridge between Heart and Kidneys. The Heart represents our spirit and our higher purpose in life, whereas the Kidneys relate more to our walk through life—our overall vitality as well as the choices we make that enable us to live out that purpose.

Often a disconnect can develop between these two aspects of the self. We may make decisions that betray our higher calling due to fear, doubt, and past pain. We then create stories to validate the reasons why we made those choices. We often have a different storyline for each of the aspects of our lives, what we've referred to before as the Nine Palaces: Career, Relationship, Health, Wealth, Home, Children, Travel, Wisdom, and Prosperity. Essentially, the stories we create revolve around the pain that we feel as it relates to each of these palaces. Taken together, they are called the Nine Heart Pains. They represent the hurts we experienced when we strayed from our Dao or our true path—the relationships lost, the wrong turns taken, the chances not seized.

In treatment, Ghost Cave brings these stories to the surface. This allows us to examine, understand, and rewrite the narratives that limit and disempower us. By reconnecting Heart and Kidneys, we can reclaim our path. The Pericardium meridian serves as the intermediary, allowing this reconnection to occur. In this way, Ghost Cave helps transmute our autobiographies from tales of "what might have been" to declarations of what we will yet become. That story's ending is still unwritten.

Indications

This point addresses symptoms related to the blood in general.

Heart pains and strife often stem from our inability to fulfill our deepest desires. When our desires continuously elude us, we can develop what Chinese Medicine calls "heat in the Heart" or "heat in the blood."

Heat in the Heart is no small matter because when there is Heart heat, the spirit becomes unsettled, which then causes many types of symptoms. For example, a person might feel isolated or ostracized from their family or their community. Or, they might simply feel that the joy has been taken out of life.

If the situation continues, a person may develop more serious emotional instability—including mania and paranoia—and many more serious signs of both mental and physical illness, as follows:

Mental illness: instability, paranoia, aggressiveness, extreme fear of the dark, self-injury or suicide attempts to get attention and be rescued, feeling upset by everything, hitting one's head against the wall, jumping around erratically, being unable to stop moving and fidgeting, continuous hand-wringing, behaving like a caged animal, needing everyone to physically back off, inappropriate laughing and giggling, amnesia caused by the ghost consuming the brain and memories, bipolar disorder (manic depression), the compulsion to hit things all the time, hibernating and avoiding social contact, or appearing to be catatonic.

Heart symptoms: Because this point is related to the heart of the heart, other symptoms may include: clogged arteries, heart palpitations, feeling heartbroken, being mean-spirited, feeling a lack of vitality, feeling like the heart is not free and the spirit is obstructed, being weighed down by memories of the past, and other symptoms related to a lack of blood flow or what we call blood stasis.

Trauma history: Ghost Cave is particularly indicated for any trauma in the person's history, including violence, sexual abuse, isolation, bullying, and ostracization.

Sensitivities: The person may be overly sensitive, or have an aversion to bright lights, crowds, or other people.

Sleep: Often when the heart and spirit are disturbed, the person can't sleep and feels exhausted. There may be sleepwalking, a refusal to sleep, or the person may complain that their eyes are wide open at night.

Heat: Because of the heat in the body, there is typically more gum disease, perhaps some bloody stools, bloody urine, or nosebleeds, or even vomiting of undigested food or blood.

Other symptoms: These may include: numbness, asthma, pressure in the diaphragm, tight jaw and neck, loss of yin or damage to the yin, emaciation, loss of appetite, drooling or foaming of the mouth, coughing up phlegm, dark circles under the eyes or a lack of sparkle in the eyes, tremors, epilepsy, convulsions, excessive bruising, a sense of feeling beaten up, or the person may feel very cold, as if they're living in a cold cave.

Treating Ghost Cave

When used in treatment, Ghost Cave generally extinguishes wind, clears heat, and generates fluids that nourish the Lungs and the Stomach without creating phlegm or stickiness in the body. It can be used for hot flashes, feverish sweating, and what's called "empty heat."

Ghost Cave clears out the debris that has collected in the arteries and Heart—the disappointment, guilt, hurt, bitterness, and resentment. The Heart needs to be empty so that the blood, which contains the spirit, can flow through it.

This point also works on helping the person let go of any paranoia, self-hatred, and self destructiveness so that both the blood and the spirit can flow freely again.

Needling: 2-5 fen (.2 to .5 cun) Many people find this point painful when needled. This may be because of the heart pain that the point is accessing. The non-needle technique allows this point to be "needled" painlessly, so that you can focus on the true underlying emotional pain, rather than the physical pain.

Energetic Approach: Vibrate this point energetically about ½ inch below the surface while focusing your attention on the person's heart.

Alternate Point: Pericardium 5 is also a similar ghost point (not one of the Ghost Points mentioned in Sun SiMiao's Ode, but one of the original set of 20 Ghost Points) that can be used alternatively and needled 2–5 fen.

Ghost Cave Self-Cultivation

This point's original name was the Palace of Nourishment, meaning that it was a point for cultivating the sense of nourishment in a person.

The most common name for the point is the Palace of Weariness or Palace of Taxation, which points out that when we do not have enough nourishment or we overdo things, we feel exhausted.

While you may think of nourishment as being related to the Earth Element and the Stomach and Spleen in Chinese Medicine, this point represents the ways you nourish your spirit, which has little to do with what you're eating or drinking. It means that true nourishment is achieved as you pursue your true passion in life. When you connect with your true passion and do things related to that passion, you will not grow weary at all. Even if the effort you're putting in is substantial and might tax another person, if it's your passion, it's not taxing to you at all. What is "work" to one person is a labor of love to another. Working at a passion is a joy that feeds the soul rather than drains it.

The first step in cultivating this point is to evaluate whether you have heart pains, which most of us do. What are the things that are being stored in your heart and causing your heart to be obstructed? Take some time to journal about them and understand them. Where did they come from? We often hang onto these pains in an effort to protect against similar events ever happening again in the future. What are you still hanging onto?

The next step is to understand what makes you feel passionate about life. If you don't already know what that is, spend some time thinking about activities and aspects of your life that make you feel the most free and connected. And if you do know what you are passionate about doing, even if you haven't been able to do it yet, explore it more fully. Take some time to journal about this... What makes you (or would make you) want to jump out of bed in the morning, ready for the day? How might you be able to allow yourself to pursue that passion even if it's not "logical" to those around you (or even to yourself)?

Ghost Cave Meditation

The goal of this meditation is to center within your truth in the cave of your heart and release any heart pains you've stored in there. The cave of your heart is the empty space inside your heart where the blood flows through—the space that holds your heart pain stories that you've created about your past trauma and negative experiences in this lifetime.

When you start to center within your truth in the center of your heart, you can begin to release your prejudices and judgments and see what that truth really is. Even if you don't like what you see, at least you will begin to see what's really there.

You can begin by finding a quiet space and having your journal or notebook next to you for recording your reflections after the meditation. Then follow the *Relax Your Body and Clear Your Mind Meditation* on page 54 of this book. You can listen to the free guided meditation in the AlchemyLearningCenter.com.

Once you are relaxed, take a few moments to clear your mind of any thoughts that arise. Now you are ready to start the Ghost Cave meditation.

Take a moment to more deeply quiet your mind, and then begin to quiet your heart. If any mental tension exists in you, let it go... Take all the to-do lists and the worries and just let them go.

Turn your attention to the center of your heart. Your heart is beating... pulsing blood and life through every cell of your body. Your heart is strong and true and it has a purpose—it circulates the life force through your body. But it does even more than that—so much more. Imagine your physical heart as a literal cave inside your chest. Imagine that you're standing outside the cave, and then begin to walk inside that cave—your very own heart cave. As you walk slowly inside, your eyes begin to adjust to the darkness. You begin to look around your cave and see what's there. What do you see? What is inside your cave?

What big, dusty, old pieces of furniture are there? Those are your old stories that perhaps you've been storing in your heart for years, or even decades.

Are there stories or pieces of furniture in your cave that you've hung onto for sentimental reasons? Are you hanging onto them because they were learning experiences? Or is it simply because you can't let them go?

Look around your inner cave. What are the memories and things from the past that are like the old dusty furniture in there. Can you pick one to look at today? Just one. What stands out to you?

Consider why you still cling to this story or object. What does it symbolize about you? What is behind it?

What is the story you're telling yourself about it? What parts of the story might not even be true? Maybe the truth of the story is broader than the more limited scope of how you tell it to yourself.

Maybe you don't even remember all the circumstances of the story. So as you re-examine this story now, what are the feelings that are coming up for you right now?

Can you center within the truth of your heart and look again at this one story you've created? What is the absolute truth about it? Try to feel for the unbiased, unprejudiced truth.

As you center within the truth of your heart, can you release this story and move that old, dusty piece of furniture out of your cave? Can you give it to the Divine Universal Garage Sale where there's more than enough room for everything? No one else cares or minds if you move it out of your cave. What has been holding you back from releasing it?

Maybe what was holding you back was that the story is so upsetting that you feel like you have to hold onto it to make sure that it never happens again.

Or maybe you're hanging onto it because there was something wonderful in the past that you're constantly longing to recreate. So you want to keep the memory alive.

Or maybe it was so traumatic, you just never stopped thinking about it. Maybe you obsessively return to thinking about it and trying to figure out why it happened.

Whatever the reason, ask yourself: Am I willing to let this go now? Is it really useful to keep it? Does this story serve me today?

If you're willing to let go of it, imagine yourself moving it outside the cave and letting the Divine Universal Garage Sale Coordinator dispose of it for you. It's moving out day. And you don't have to worry about it. Let it go.

Now that you've removed it from your cave, go back into the cave and feel the new energy inside your heart with some new open space inside. There's more room to breathe and to feel. It's a little more spacious inside your heart. How does that feel? What feelings are coming up for you here and now?

When you're finished, you can slowly open your eyes and see the present moment around you. Write your thoughts and feelings in your journal.

You can listen to this guided meditation at the Alchemy Learning Center (AlchemyLearningCenter.com).

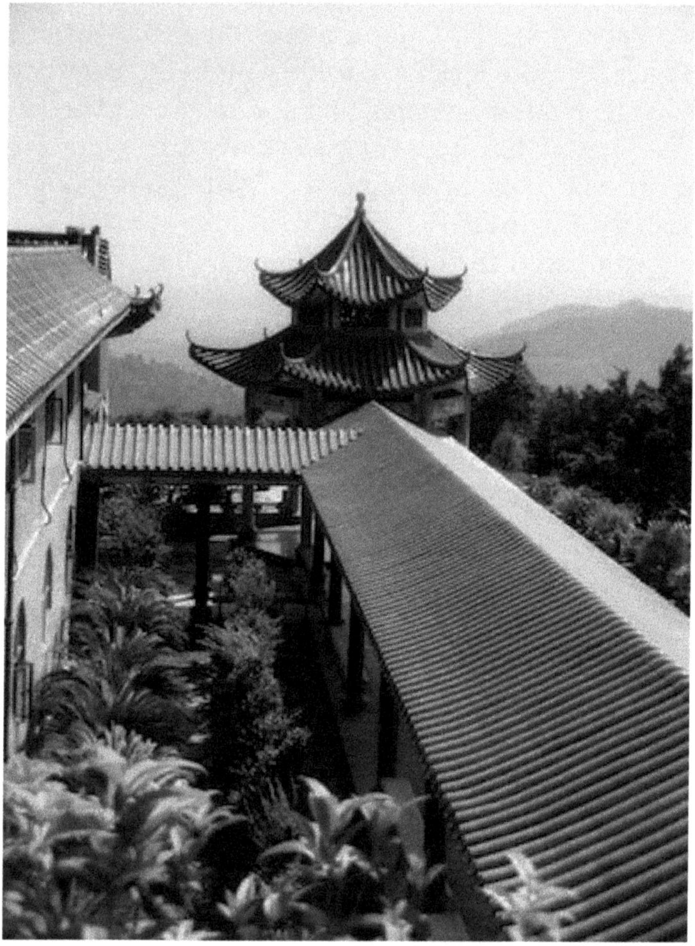

Huanglong Temple, LuoFu Shan (Ge Hong's mountain), Huizhou, China

The Fourth Trinity of the Ghost Points – Your Identity

The Fourth Trinity is really a trinity plus one extra point (the 13th point). Thirteen is a very important number in Chinese numerology. It's called the number of Disillusionment… which indicates the moment when a person comes to realize that life is just an illusion.

The first two Trinities summon up the presence of yang in the body. The Third Trinity restores yin, by creating fluids such as saliva. In this Trinity, the person is losing yang completely, so we have to safeguard what yang is left, and then consolidate the *Jing*/Essences.

This trinity addresses the deepest, darkest issues that come from experiencing trauma and other negative experiences, and from getting hooked by "ghosts" of all sorts. So if the person hasn't spoken about their trauma yet (many people hesitate to share these dark stories), it often comes out in this trinity.

Specifically, the points in this trinity deal with guilt and shame, betrayal, abuse, oppression, and severe trauma. Here we're dealing with trauma that is severe enough to cut you off from your core identity. In theory, mild cases of emotional blocks may not need a practitioner to do the Fourth Trinity or even the entire Thirteen Ghost Point protocol, as we have said before. However, we typically find it useful to do the entire protocol even with people who don't have this level of trauma. In this case, the last points are an amazing exploration of the person's spiritual growth overall. You can think of it as a way of exploring the person's relationship with Heaven (Du 23), Earth (Ren 1), Humanity (LI 11) and with the last point, the root of all that is (the point at the root of the tongue).

At this point in the progression of the Thirteen Ghost Points, yin and yang have separated, bringing about "vexation and agitation" or even collapse or loss of consciousness. If the ghost has progressed this far, it is consuming the yin and the yang and may be causing severe mental disorders. The person may act as if they're someone else. Symptoms overall are much more severe, including fragile skin that looks bruised or scarred, being emotionally and mentally overwhelmed, being unable to control bodily functions, shaking uncontrollably, speaking in tongues, and being mentally deranged. While these symptoms are quite severe, we've found that many people who have none of these symptoms also benefit from these points because they address themes like guilt, shame, and oppression.

This trinity attempts to safeguard and consolidate the *Jing*/Essences to stop any further damage to them.

10 Ghost Hall – Gui Tang, Du 23

The character used for the word Hall is not the great hall at the entrance of the palace where you would greet strangers. This Hall is a room next to your heart—in the inner sanctum of your palace—a Hall where you receive only the most trusted people in your life. These are your most intimate companions. The hope is that these people won't poison you or stab you in the back.

If you've been emotionally stabbed in the back before or have experienced abuse or some other horrible trauma, it may be difficult to trust anyone anymore, even the ones who actually are the most trustworthy. Intimacy might be nearly impossible. You might feel like you're never going to let anyone in again. Even love is not worth the risk.

In fact, you might not be letting yourself into your own heart. You may have walled it off so that it's as if there is a cellophane wrapper around it and no one can get through, not even you!

You've done this because in your story about the experience, you have blamed yourself. If you were violated, how did you make the mistake to trust the person who hurt you to begin with? The questions of blame go on. How did you allow yourself to be violated? And how can you trust that there are good people out there? How can you trust yourself to be the judge of that? How can you trust the Divine to keep you safe?

There are so many levels of trust that you're dealing with. And in grappling with it, the "ghost" is consuming your energy —both yin and yang. Contamination is causing the consumption of the *Jing*/Essences, burning up both yin and yang and phlegm is blocking internal pathways. This contamination can even be coming from your own mental state —where you are essentially contaminating yourself.

This point in combination with Ren 1 (the next Ghost point) represents the foundation of yin and yang. Du 23, *Shang*

Xing, or the Upper Star, is the highest point on the body and the *Du Mai* vessel.[19] So we're trying to safeguard what yang is left in the upper body and the head with the most yang point, and then utilize the lowest point of the body, Ren 1, *Hui Yin*, or the Meeting of Yin, which is the most yin point, to restore the yin. Used together we're consolidating the *Jing* both above and below.

The Upper Star represents the North Star, the constant star around which all the other stars orbit. It's the constancy of you that is the part you can trust. You may have been thrown off course by betrayal or trauma, but there's still something constant in you that will never change—your spirit. We want to consolidate and support the constancy of who you are as opposed to the derailment you experienced after a painful event.

This point allows a person to realign with the stars, with the light, with the heavens, with something astral or stellar, and it brings that stellar connection into your consciousness. You are receiving and reconnecting to your guidance that you lost after experiencing the betrayal or trauma.

Indications

The heat is raging and has become empty heat due to the yin depletion.

While the following symptoms are much more severe, many people with few symptoms still have intimacy issues and may benefit from this point as part of the whole protocol.

Severe mental illness: There are many symptoms and conditions associated with this point: effects on the Shen/ spirit in the brain, raging heat, mania, vexation and agitation, dementia, dissociative disorders, Alzheimer's disease caused by

---

[19] The *Du Mai* is one of the Eight Extraordinary Vessels that runs from the tailbone, over the top of head, and down to the top lip (Du 26 - Ghost Palace, the first Ghost Point.)

phlegm blocking the internal pathways, stone cold depression even to the point of collapse and loss of consciousness, eating dirt or fecal excrements, contaminating oneself, and suicide. Intermittent signs and symptoms with heat include: tremors, shaking, progressive neurological diseases, more frequent and intense memory lapses, loss of motor activity, multiple sclerosis, numbness, neuropathy, forgetting how to walk, and being unable to feed oneself.

Other symptoms: Nasal congestion, poor vision, and dizzy spells.

Treating Ghost Hall

Treating Du 23 brings in the light, opens nasal passages, and relaxes the jaw.

Needling: Traditionally this was needled 3–5 fen (.3 to .5 cun).

Energetic Approach: Placing your finger on the point, allow the energy to "needle" into the skull about 3–5 fen.

Moxibustion: You can add moxibustion to bring in more light, for example when the treatment hasn't yet brought light back into their eyes.

Ghost Hall Self-Cultivation

Cultivating this point returns access to yourself when it's been blocked. Not having access to yourself means you cannot even be in an intimate relationship with yourself, let alone with others. Are you able and willing to access your deepest self?

This point helps you begin to trust others again if your trust has previously been violated. Using it can provide answers to some of the most difficult questions. How are you going to trust again? Are you able to feel safe exposing your most vulnerable parts with a trusted person? How are you going to let anyone into your inner sanctum? How can you trust yourself to know who is safe if you failed to have good judgment in the past?

As the highest point on the body, Ghost Hall also represents the alignment with the stars and specifically with a person's North Star... the star that guides us if we're ever lost in the world. If something is taking you over, your North Star points the direction to your authentic self. Ghost Hall brings the astral, the light of heaven, the stellar into your consciousness. Can you align yourself with the stars and the light of heaven? Can you allow the stellar to come into your consciousness?

What is your North Star—the thing that is constant in your life? Do you have something internal that is constant or are you governed and even ruled by others?

Du 23 is followed by Ren 1, the lowest point on the torso. As above, so below. The movement is bringing the light down from heaven into the darkness below. Can you turn on the light in your own darkness?

Another way to cultivate this point is through Stone Medicine. Master Jeffrey Yuen gave a suggestion to try Golden Stellar Calcite (sometimes known as Dogtooth Calcite or Stellar Beam Calcite), which is an Alchemical stone that is in the process of transforming itself (it's almost transparent).

You can place this stone on the point, so it acts like an antenna pointing to the stars. The idea is that the stone will help you capture the astral energy and vibrations. It also calms the spirit and evokes divine presence, which then stops the *Jing*/Essences from being contaminated. Oyster shell can be used as a substitute for Golden Stellar Calcite, which can sometimes be hard to find or very expensive.

Ghost Hall Meditation

The goal of this meditation is to feel safe enough to open up to a greater sense of intimacy in your life.

You can begin by finding a quiet space and having your journal or notebook next to you for recording your reflections after the meditation. Then follow the *Relax Your Body and Clear Your Mind Meditation* on page 54 of this book. You can listen to the free guided meditation in the AlchemyLearningCenter.com.

Once you are relaxed, take a few moments to clear your mind of any thoughts that arise. Now you are ready to start the Ghost Hall meditation.

Bring your attention to the center of your heart. In this meditation you are the sovereign ruler within your own palace. You get to decide everything in this space, regardless of the outcome. In this palace, your bedroom (which is the center of your heart) is a sacred part of your palace where only the safest people are allowed. Outside of this innermost sanctum is a small hall, an antechamber room, where you receive only the safest guests. These are the guests who you feel you can trust implicitly and allow to get close to your heart. They aren't going to betray you, poison you, or stab you in the back—emotionally or otherwise. You can be and feel safe in this space with those people who you allow into this sacred space.

Let's imagine you are sitting quietly alone in your inner sanctum space, the space you just imagined. In this room, you can be intimate with people you can trust and it feels good to you to be there. Just sit for a moment and be in the safety of that room, the center of your heart. Feel how safe it is when you're there alone.

If you don't feel safe, that's perfectly okay. Some people do not feel safe inside their hearts. This meditation will help. Just do your best to feel as calm as you can in the center of your heart, your inner sanctum inside the palace of your body.

Now ask yourself: Who is safe to let into my room? Do you ever let anyone into this room? Can you trust anyone at all? Do you know or have any safe people in your life right now?

Do you have a lot of fear? Are you afraid to let anyone into this room? Can anyone get close to you on a deep and intimate level?

If the feeling is yes or if the answer is no… ask yourself why this is. Why does it feel okay to let certain people in? And why do you feel afraid to let other types of people in?

If you do feel fear, it may be because you don't know how to tell whether people are safe. Perhaps you're not sure how to recognize when someone is unsafe.

If you've been fooled or betrayed before, how can you ever trust anyone again? Can you even trust yourself and your own judgment?

What feelings are coming up for you at this moment? Fear, anger, sadness, loneliness? Are there any feelings? Take a few moments to look at what has arisen in your thoughts right now.

The universal truth for all living beings is that no one is completely safe in the world. As humans, we need to sometimes choose to do things that are selfish or can be perceived as selfish to others, which means sometimes we end up hurting our loved ones, even if we don't mean to.

Can you imagine letting someone you trust into your inner sacred space, knowing that there are no guarantees of safety? Can you trust your instincts and your true feelings? Is there more potential for good in letting this person in than there is the potential for a hurtful or painful outcome? Is Love worth the risk?

Take a few minutes now to imagine who you can or will let into your intimate antechamber, and then sit with how it feels to open your heart intimately to the true authenticity of who you are in this lifetime. If there is no one who feels safe to you at present, let the feelings flow and imagine what that person might look and feel like, or what that experience might feel like to you. Don't force it. Let it come easily if it can.

When you're ready, come back to the present moment and open your eyes. Write any thoughts or feelings that come to you in your journal.

You can listen to this guided meditation at the Alchemy Learning Center (AlchemyLearningCenter.com).

11 Ghost Hidden – Gui Cang, Ren 1 or Yu Men

This is the point of shame and guilt. Ghost Hidden is the storage place where we hide the things we're ashamed of deep down inside, trying to bury them "underground," hoping they'll disappear.

This point is in the genital area and is the lowest place on the torso. It's the meeting point of the *Ren Mai*, *Chong Mai*, and *Du Mai*,[20] which is called the First Ancestry. In this case, the Ghost wishes to destroy the ancestry, so the person may feel suicidal. Drowning was the most common way for someone to kill themself in ancient times, and Ren 1 was traditionally used if someone was drowning.

Ghost Hidden is an important point for a person who has any history of sexual abuse. Many times when a person is a victim of sexual abuse or another kind of bodily violence, they may turn on themselves and believe that it was somehow their fault. They might come to believe that they are bad people at their heart center, and they carry their shame and guilt with them always.

This point releases that shame and helps the person feel forgiven. It helps them find the part of them that knows it wasn't their fault and that they did nothing wrong.

We often draw upon the Christian parable of the Prodigal Son, a biblical story illustrating God's unconditional love for humanity. The Prodigal Son squanders his inheritance on reckless pursuits and, upon returning home penniless, expects his father to reject him for all his wrongdoings.

This point represents the Prodigal Son begging for forgiveness, kneeling at his father's doorstep, pounding his fists on the threshold, lamenting, "Father, please let me in. I know I've been so bad. Why won't you accept me?" Unaware of his father standing on the inside, lovingly inviting him to enter,

---

[20] The *Ren Mai*, *Chong Mai*, and *Du Mai* are three of the Eight Extraordinary Vessels.

the son remains fixated on his own guilt and self-condemnation.

Blinded by his own negative self-perception, he fails to recognize that he is already forgiven. His father is celebrating his return, as if there were nothing to forgive. Eventually, the Prodigal Son is reunited with his father, and in a sense, with himself.

As in this parable, the guilt or yin aspect converges with forgiveness or yang aspect at this point. So in treating this point, we're trying to consolidate the remaining yin in the body, because the "ghost" has been eating up the yin. When you lose much of your yin and yang energy, it causes a separation that brings on depression and even suicidal tendencies. This point is attempting to bring them back together by consolidating the Jing/Essences.

Indications

While this point's signs and symptoms are much more severe than those of the other Trinities, many people with few symptoms may still have a lot of guilt and shame that has accumulated over their years of life. Many people benefit from this point as part of the whole protocol.

Emotional: Shame and embarrassment, wanting to hide from the world, feeling as if one is actually drowning.

Mental Illness: Bipolar disorder, mania caused by excessive heat, serious suicidal feelings and attempts that are now more likely to succeed, and doing risky things to invite death.

Physical symptoms: Vaginal protrusions, vaginal pain, prolapse, menstrual issues, incontinence.

Treating Ghost Hidden

Ghost Hidden consolidates yin and yang energy in the body. It also strengthens the lower back, regulates the *Chong Mai* and *Ren Mai*, clears heat, and releases the lower orifices so that unwanted things can be purged.

Ghost Hidden has two point locations depending on the genital anatomy of a person.

For individuals born with external or penile genital anatomy the point is Ren 1, located at the perineum, halfway between the scrotum and the anus.

For persons born with internal or vulvic genital anatomy, the point is Yu Men that is located halfway between the clitoris and where the top of the labia parts.

We cannot assume what anatomy a person has, even with cisgender clients. Therefore it is important to respectfully ask what a person would like their body parts to be called and to explain the options for the types of treatments they can receive. This is especially important when working with gender-diverse, gender non-conforming, transwomen, transmen, and intersex clients.

For example, transmasculine people may wish to have Ren 1 treated, or for transfeminine clients, an energetic Yu Men treatment may be more helpful and gender affirming. Also, consider doing both points.

These points are not needled in the treatment. Instead they are traditionally warmed with a small moxa stick. The moxa is an important component to the healing, especially for anyone who has experienced sexual abuse in the past, because it brings warmth and yang energy to an area that has been injured and possibly shut down for a long time.

This requires much conscientiousness and in-person training to do properly and to ensure safety, both physically and emotionally. It requires the client to help hold the genitals in a position that allows for the moxibustion technique to get close but not touch the area.

Because these points can be difficult for some clients to have treated, it's important to have a discussion with them before doing this point. In many cases, they may be uncomfortable doing this point and you will need an alternate technique.

Energetic Approach: You can do this point energetically without the moxa. Or you can use one of the alternate points. To do this point energetically, hover the palm of your hand (PC 8) over the point. Place your other hand on the Ren 2 area to connect with the Ren Mai channel. Treat the point energetically, as if you're doing a long-distance treatment, using energy from your PC 8 point on your palm as "the needle."

Alternate Points: When using an alternate point, use your intention and focus on the principles of Ghost Hidden when doing the point.

One option for alternate points is the extra point, PC 7.5 (Daling/Great Heart), located on the base of the palm, 1 cun distal to PC 7. This is a Korean hand acupuncture point for Ren 1.

Another alternate point for Ren 1 is Du 26 in facial reflexology. However, since this is another Ghost Point, it may not serve as the best substitute.

Ghost Hidden Cultivation

Many of us have experienced times in our lives where our spirit feels lost or deadened. Often in these instances, we feel a deep loss of energy and a sense of utter exhaustion. That's because it is only when the spirit infuses the blood that our qi can flow. We need adequate blood to have proper qi flow.

What will resuscitate your spirit at times like these when all feels lost?

The answer is: **You** will! This point helps you to embrace your perfection and your self-forgiveness. You are perfect, not wrong or broken. In fact, this point is about your return to innocence. What would it take for you to return to the state of innocence that you were born in?

This may also mean that it's time to speak up for yourself in the world and stop hiding. It's time to tell your true story without shame. How do you want to reframe and retell your story? And if you do, who will you tell it to?

Case Study: Face-to-Face with the Past Perpetrator

During her Ghost Points treatment, one woman told her story of a date rape that occurred during her teenage years. The person who did this to her was not only a part of her community, but a friend of her family's. She had never told anyone about it because she felt like she'd done something wrong to make him think it was okay to force her into having sex. She was the one who held the shame of the experience.

After her Ghost Points treatment, she returned home and confronted him. She needed to reclaim her voice and assert her truth—that what he did was unequivocally wrong. After that, the relentless grip of obsessive thoughts about past events finally ceased, allowing her to break free and embrace the present.

Before the treatment, the scars of her past had made navigating romantic relationships a daunting task. After she confronted the abuser and liberated herself from the burden of shame, a remarkable shift happened. She found herself open to love and creating meaningful connections. She ultimately found her way to a long-lasting and healthy partnership.

Once shame is lifted, a person often feels empowered to do what's right for them, whether that means confronting wrongdoers, seeking justice, or simply moving forward with their life. The point isn't what action they take but that they now have the freedom to do whatever they need to do.

Ghost Hidden Meditation

This meditation adds to the previous Divine Concierge Meditation for Ghost Bed. In this meditation, you can try to identify any guilt or shame you may have in your mind, allowing yourself to release it to the Divine Concierge, and then this time, you will actually enter the white light, which represents Divine unconditional acceptance.

You can begin by finding a quiet space and having your journal or notebook next to you for recording your reflections after the meditation. Then follow the *Relax Your Body and Clear Your Mind Meditation* on page 54 of this book. You may listen to the guided meditation at the AlchemyLearningCenter.com.

Once you are relaxed, take a few moments to clear your mind of any thoughts that arise. Now you are ready to start the Ghost Hidden meditation.

Imagine you are in a large, sparsely furnished room, empty except for a round table in the center of the room. The back wall is one huge, open doorway emanating a brilliant beautiful white light. Imagine that this wall of light is an entrance to the Divine. Now bring your attention back to the empty table. This table will be where you are going to place all the guilt and shame that you have been carrying in your "emotional backpack."

As you calmly enter this room, ask yourself these questions: Do I have any guilt or shame that I hold deep down inside of myself? What do I feel guilty about in my life? Do I have a memory of a shaming event? Was I shamed by someone else? Or was I the one who shamed another person? What happened in the past that caused me to have those feelings?

These are the negative feelings that you keep in your emotional backpack, which now feels so heavy on your shoulders. Can you feel it?

Standing at the table in the center of the room, reach behind you and slide off your backpack and open it so you can look inside.

Gently remove the guilt or shame from your backpack and place it on the table in front of you. It can be one or many items.

You are giving it over to your personal Divine Manager, your spiritual concierge, to purge it for you. The Divine Concierge is happy to be there to serve you and take care of your problems, your challenging issues, your old stories, and even your complaints. Simply place on the table any feelings you have been carrying that make you feel guilty, shameful, tainted, or not worthy of Divine love. And don't worry—there is an endless amount of room on the table.

As you place each burden on the table, one by one, release it and let it go. With each burden released, you begin to once again experience the innocence of the day you were born. You will feel lighter and lighter with each story you remove from the backpack and place on the table.

Now that you've released your guilt and shame and the rebellious qi that went with them, you can slowly turn and face the expansive doorway of white light. Slowly begin to walk into the light, freely and effortlessly. You are walking directly into the light of the Divine.

As you step into the light, you can feel the total acceptance of Divine love recognizing the perfection of you. There is nothing wrong or bad about you. You can release anything bad that was said to you, and whatever that story was, it is now simply dissolving in truth. You are good and worthy of Divine love. You can feel this sense of love wash over you.

When you're ready, you can come back to the room with the round table.

Here you have a choice. If you leave the items you placed on the table, your Divine Manager, your Spiritual Concierge, will take care of them. You can now leave everything behind and trust that it will be resolved. All will be well. On the other hand, if you're not ready to fully let go of your guilt and shame stories, you don't have to! You can pick them up from the table. For example, you may feel you need to make amends for something you feel guilty about before you let it go. Sometimes it takes several attempts before you can trust that you can let them go.

When you're ready, you can open your eyes and come back to the present moment.

You can listen to this guided meditation at the Alchemy Learning Center (AlchemyLearningCenter.com).

12 Ghost Official/Leg/Burial – Gui Chen, Large Intestine 11

We all have many rules in our lives, some societal, some familial, and some that we develop from our own personal beliefs and values.

Humans create rules that are generally based on their values, morals, ethics, and religious beliefs. We decide, as a species, for the most part, that there are specific requirements for how we want to live our lives based on these beliefs. The rules tend to dictate how we want to live out our values and indicate what's most important about what we believe. People follow rules in order to fulfill those individual or group values.

Childhood is typically a time when we have to play by other people's rules. Some of us are given choices about how we want to live, and our parents, teachers, and elders encourage us to discover who we want to be and how we want to behave. In fact, these days, we are often encouraged to allow our will to create our own destiny.

But many children face oppression from their caregivers and their rules. Once they grow up, they should be capable of making their own choices, but they might still hear the old voices from their upbringing echoing in their minds, leading to self-oppression.

One example of societal rules from the Judeo-Christian tradition is the Ten Commandments, which include instructions like, "Thou shalt not kill." Many societal laws are designed around religious tenets such as these.

Some individuals expand upon the societal belief system, and, for example, decide that killing animals is also sinful. They might become vegetarian or vegan in order to live according to those rules. And while it's not illegal to cheat on your spouse, many people live by the rule based on the commandment, "Thou shalt not commit adultery."

However, these rules don't need to be tied to religious precepts. An individual's rules might be as simple as always being kind to others, or always telling the truth, or always giving someone the benefit of the doubt when things are uncertain. These are just a few of the many personal rules that we may or may not choose to live by.

Large Intestine 11 is a Metal point, which is fundamentally about the determination of what is right and what is wrong or, as some might say, morality. What is the essence of your morality? And are you living according to what you believe is right?

This point asks us: Who is in charge of your being? Are you calling the shots or is someone else oppressing you?

Are you able to live by your rules, or do you feel oppressed by the rules of others? Does life seem unfair? Are you constantly beaten down? Do you lack any power and feel unable to be yourself because of society's rules or some other obstacle to your sense of fairness?

An alternate name for this point is Ghost Leg. This refers back to the explanation of Ghost Road. Are you able to walk your road in life? You cannot walk your road if your will is not your own. Ghost Leg represents a deeper version of why you might find it difficult to walk your road. Ghost Road focuses more on the distractions and fears within yourself that may be keeping you from walking your destiny. Ghost Leg embodies the much more challenging concept that now your legs are not your own. Have you been subjugated to the rules of an oppressive force in your life? Are you walking your life the way you want to?

Indications

A person needs this point when they feel very stuck in life and cannot move forward. Their will to do anything is completely absent. They may have a lot of ideas about what they want to do, but they simply cannot implement any of them. It's as if someone else (the "ghost") is running the show.

Often, when inquiring into the person's past, you may find that there was an oppressive parent or elder who disempowered them on a regular basis. Or sometimes a person may have experienced this in a relationship as an adult with a powerful, abusive partner.

Paired with Ghost Road, this point helps get to the deeper reasons why someone cannot walk their life destiny's road.

Classical symptoms may include:

Heat: Empty heat lingering in the head that may be causing mental illness, high or intermittent fevers, being suicidal, the inability to interact with others, "demonic" or cruel and harmful behavior, or self-harming.

Physical symptoms: The person may be black and blue around the crease of the elbow (Large Intestine 11), may look beaten up, or their platelet count may be off. They may be experiencing vomiting, edema, or frequent infections (pestilent qi), neuropathy (especially in the legs) or even falling into a coma. They may feel as if they are no longer having communication with the outside world (in an introverted state of yin) and don't have a place in society. They may stop eating or be emaciated.

Treating Ghost Official

Recovering someone's will who has been oppressed isn't just about removing the oppressor. At this stage, the oppressed person also has to go through a transformational process that will allow them to find themselves again. Because this point has to clear away something that has been blocked for perhaps a very long time, the point needs additional stimulation in light of the fact that so much yang qi has been lost.

The Fire Mountain Needle technique, which was also used on Ghost Road, the 5th point, provides the extra heat and yang qi. Additional manipulation of the needle is also helpful.

See *Treating Ghost Road* on page 159 for more information on both the needling and energetic techniques for this point.

This point clears the lingering, raging empty heat, especially in the head.

Ghost Official Self-Cultivation

Your spirit gets to live by your own rules. You do not have to be subjugated by other people's oppression. You get to have the choice of obeying various societal rules or creating your own rules to live by.

What are the rules you live by currently and have lived by in the past? How many rules have you made for yourself in your lifetime and how many rules were given to you?

Create three columns on a piece of paper.

- In the first column, write down a list of the rules you are currently living by.
- In the second column, write down where the rule came from, whether it was yourself, another person, society, or your religious upbringing.
- In the third column, write yes or no: Yes, I want to continue to live by this rule or No, I don't want to live by this rule anymore.

Now, review the list. What rules are missing? If you can create whatever rules you want to live by (and then actually live by them), what would they be?

Now make a new list that can incorporate the rules you want to keep from the previous list and add to them.

The Ghost Official point oversees our beliefs. A rule can be a procedure you follow, but it can also be a commandment to the universe. For example, "I am healthy" is an affirmation, but if you live by the rule that "I am healthy," it becomes a commandment to the universe. By committing to this rule, you won't entertain thoughts of ill health, even if you experience pain or symptoms. This type of commandment changes the very structure of your thinking and leaves no room for doubt. Another example is the affirmation, "I am lovable." As a commandment, "I am lovable" takes on a much greater power. If someone expresses hatred towards you, you won't take it personally because you live by the rule that you are lovable. This perspective allows you to see their pain as a reflection of their own issues, not a judgment of your worth.

Write down any rules you wish to create. Make sure that you feel the desire to commit to living by them. This may be difficult. At first it may seem like a wish list and not feasible.

The next level of cultivation is making a commitment to yourself to live by your own rules.

It may take some time. You may have to spend a good bit of time contemplating what life would be like living by these new rules before you can commit to them. How will your life change when you embrace living by your own rules?

Ghost Official Meditation

In this meditation, you will explore and discover your own life rules. Today, in a kind, loving, and non-judgmental way, you will examine whether you've been able to live by your own rules in your life. Have you lived by them in the past? Are you living by them in the present time? How will you live in the future? This is also a writing exercise, so be prepared to write down any feelings or thoughts that may arise from this meditation.

This meditation is a gentle exploration to cultivate awareness of where you are in your life and where you have been in your life with no judgment of good or bad, right or wrong... just a loving and compassionate assessment of how you are moving in the world today.

You can begin by finding a quiet space and having your journal or notebook next to you for recording your reflections after the meditation. Then follow the *Relax Your Body and Clear*

Your Mind Meditation on page 54 of this book. You can listen to the free guided meditation in the AlchemyLearningCenter.com.

Once you are relaxed, take a few moments to clear your mind of any thoughts that arise. Now you are ready to start the Ghost Official meditation.

Now let's begin by revisiting your early childhood years for a moment. Reflect on your formative years growing up.

Were you encouraged to seek your own destiny and manifest your own will, or were you expected or forced to follow other people's rules that you disagreed with? If you were able to manifest your own destiny and have your own rules, what rules did you create for yourself? If you were oppressed and unable to manifest your own destiny or create your own rules, what rules did you wish to live by then? Did the rules you were living by make you happy and content or was there a feeling of conflict inside of yourself?

Now turn your attention back to your current day life and how you live your life. How many of your current rules are truly aligned with how you want to live your life? How many of them are someone else's rules? Are you in harmony or conflict with the rules you live by?

How do you think you should be living your life? Would you change any rules you live by if you had the choice? If so, how? What new rules would you want to embrace?

Select one new rule you would like to incorporate into your life. Remember what it means to live by a rule that is undeniable and maybe even immutable for you. Can you make that level of commitment to yourself to live by this rule and not doubt it? Embracing the rule should feel like a relief not a burden. If it's a burden, then it's probably something from someone else's belief system, not part of your true beliefs.

When you're ready, you can open your eyes and come back to the present moment. Write your feelings and thoughts in your journal.

You can listen to this guided meditation at the Alchemy Learning Center (AlchemyLearningCenter.com).

13 Ghost Seal – *Gui Feng, Hai Quan or Yin Tang*

The word Seal represents your core identity, your incarnation in this lifetime, your soul when it first incarnated—the truest essence of you. This point clears the soul of any contamination it may have accumulated.

In the old days, when people sealed a letter, they melted wax over the fold and pressed a stamp with their insignia into the wax to verify the identity of the sender and as a way to ensure the recipient that the letter had not been tampered with.

The question is: Who are you at a very fundamental level? What would be your insignia or the image that undeniably represents who you are?

Has the ghost completely changed your identity, so that you don't even recognize yourself anymore?

Treating the Ghost Seal point becomes necessary when the "ghost" completely takes over a person's soul, sealing their fate. Suicide attempts made now will be much more likely to succeed.

Indications

In severe cases, this point represents a complete takeover by the "ghost," which is now depleting the Jing/Essences of the body.

However, as part of the entire protocol, many people with few symptoms will also benefit from this point, although it may be difficult for them to articulate how or why except that they feel very calm and connected.

Physical Symptoms: The person may experience total exhaustion or look beaten and black and blue all over, as if the "ghost" is hitting them from inside (*Hai* means hurt). The skin may be peeling off. There may be many infections or fevers due to heat in the blood. The person may feel suicidal, or they may simply look like they want to die.

Mental illness: The person may seem very disturbed, be hysterical, have violent episodes, have severe psychosis or schizophrenia.

Treating Ghost Seal

Hai Quan is an extra point on the bottom of the tongue. It's located halfway between the tip and base of the tongue. Some practitioners locate it further back in the center of the underside of the tongue at the base of the frenulum. However, in ancient times, this point was needled all the way through the tongue, which might indicate that the first position in the middle of the tongue was likely the one used.

This point requires much conscientiousness and in-person training to do properly, in order to ensure safety, both physically and emotionally. It requires the patient to put their tongue on the roof of their mouth while the point is needled, and then the needle is retained and held between the front teeth. When the needle is removed, there is some bleeding, and sometimes the whole tongue changes color for a moment. It is a very daunting technique, and thankfully, there is a non-needling technique that we encourage all of our students to use.

This point is interesting because it's the one point in the treatment when the client truly can't speak. Even with Du 26, a person can speak, though it is a bit difficult. A thought to consider here is that modern day tongue piercings could essentially be thought of as a Ghost Point treatment.

Since at this point the ghost may be consuming your physical essences, your body desperately needs more yin to survive. This point is replenishing the yin by increasing salivation. Saliva is a form of yin.

Energetic Approach: You can do this point energetically by vibrating your finger on the point. Or you can use an alternate point (see below). Sitting behind the person, place your index finger on the center of the bottom of the tongue.

Let the person rest their teeth on your hand and let them swallow whenever they need to.

Alternate point: Use the extra point, Yin Tang, 2 fen, at the third eye between the eyebrows.

Case Study: Here's to You, Mrs. Robinson

A woman was referred to Leta many years ago by another practitioner. Leta had never met this client, who was hospitalized for a sudden and unexplained psychosis. She was put through a week of intense testing to determine the cause, but nothing turned up. Leta was asked to treat her in the hospital.

When Leta arrived, the woman was babbling to herself. She learned that the staff had instituted a policy of 24-hour supervision due to the woman's need to pull things off the shelves and take off her own clothes.

Leta tried to engage with her by having a conversation, but the woman was not able to converse coherently. As Leta began the treatment, the woman kept attempting to take Leta's clothes off as well, gently pulling and moving them around as Leta worked. Needless to say, it was a bit challenging at first.

Leta began playing the music she had brought with her. At that time, she had about 13,000 songs on an iPod. The treatment went on for hours but nothing was shifting. At some point, Leta began to wonder if the treatment would have any effect at all, let alone actually work. However, on the very last point, a song came on her little iPod and speaker. It was the song "Mrs. Robinson" by Simon and Garfunkel, which had the refrain: "Here's to you, Mrs. Robinson..." Once the song started, the woman looked directly at Leta, removed Leta's hand from the point on the bottom of her tongue, and said, "That's me."

Leta had only been told the woman's first name. So she didn't understand why the woman was saying that and tried to resume the treatment. But she grabbed Leta's arm again and said, "No, that's me. I'm Mrs. Robinson." It turns out that Robinson was her last name.

She had completely come back to herself. She and Leta talked for a while. She talked about her life, her battle with depression. All the signs of her psychosis were gone. She was completely coherent and was released from the hospital a few days later, completely normal. She went back to work and the life she was living beforehand as if nothing had ever happened.

Ghost Seal Self-Cultivation

To cultivate this point, you'll need to connect with the true essence of you—who you are at the core. This is the essential part of you that was you before you were even born. It's the part of you that cannot be changed in any way, even by life's traumas.

This is the immutable part of your spirit, the spirit that infuses your body with life. The spirit is always whole and cannot be broken. Only the vehicle of the spirit, which we call the body, can suffer.

Reconnecting with your spirit and wholeness in general can help the body heal, as it remembers the original blueprint of this lifetime, what this spirit came to experience. The following meditation will help you reconnect with your original spirit.

Ghost Seal Meditation

In this meditation, you will go back to the origin of you, and discover the true essence of who you really are.

You can begin by finding a quiet space and having your journal or notebook next to you for recording your reflections after the meditation. Then follow the *Relax Your Body and Clear Your Mind Meditation* on page 54 of this book. You can listen to the free guided meditation in the AlchemyLearningCenter.com.

Once you are relaxed, take a few moments to clear your mind of any thoughts that arise. Now you are ready to start the Ghost Seal meditation.

With your tongue, touch the roof of your mouth and with your forefinger touch the Ghost Seal point. If the forefinger is too uncomfortable, you can use your thumb on the point, like you're sucking your thumb. Whatever is more comfortable for you is fine, as long as you are touching the point.

Travel back in time, going backwards through your lifetime… way back to the time just before you were born, when you were a fetus, safe and warm in your mother's womb.

This space is where and when you were safely inside your mother's belly and never felt disconnected from the whole because all your needs were met by an umbilical cord that fed you. Life was good for you in your little safe, warm, gentle place.

But you left the wholeness of your mother's safe space and chose to come into this lifetime to become a separate being. Can you connect with the part of you that became separate from your mother, separate from the whole? This is the part of you that has an identity. Your own identity, like a seal or insignia (or what is called a "chop" in China) that represents you in the world. Yours and yours alone.

As you touch this point on the base of your tongue, imagine yourself as an infant nursing. You can't talk yet. This is your non-verbal time. You can only suckle and swallow.

You are in the early days of your life and creating separateness from your mother. Now you have to take action to feed yourself, when before, in the womb, you didn't have to do anything. Now you are separate from your mother, and this tongue is the vehicle for your nutrients.

If everything goes well for you after birth, your mother nurses you or another loving person feeds you, and you never go hungry. You get to experience this wonderful, beautiful nurturing as you become separate from your loving mother. You can feel connected and separate at the same time.

Or, perhaps, for you, your mother or another person who cared for you was ill or simply not a nurturing person. In fact, you had to demand what you needed through crying. Or perhaps you were ignored or even malnourished as a result.

But even so, your core identity developed, and grew over time... as you became more separate and more independent, you found ways to nourish yourself, grow and soothe yourself to get your needs met.

Imagine how you experienced the feeling of emergence from the wholeness into the separateness. If you have early childhood trauma, try to imagine the time when you were the most safe and cared for, either in the womb or outside the womb. Go to that time and space if you can find it. If you can't, try to imagine what it would be like to feel a level of safety in a womb-like environment.

Without any words, feel what it felt like to come into the world and create your separate identity in the world.

Now gently and lovingly ask yourself: Who is this being that is choosing to manifest in this lifetime?

What is my true identity?

Can I connect to my true self, my spirit?

Don't seek the answers, just allow them to come to you or gently feel into the true essence of you. For this meditation, you don't need words. There are simply feelings that can be free to surface as to who you truly are at the very core of your existence.

When you're ready, you can open your eyes and come back to the present moment. Write your feelings and thoughts in your journal.

You can listen to this guided meditation at the Alchemy Learning Center (AlchemyLearningCenter.com).

Adding Points

Typically, we wait until the follow-up treatment to add additional points when treating with the Thirteen Ghost Points. However, recognizing that each person has unique circumstances, if you feel guided to add more points into the protocol at the end of the long treatment or at the end of the last of a series of Ghost Point treatments, according to the person's specific needs, you can, of course, do so. We prefer to complete the original thirteen points before adding more in during a separate appointment to maintain a sense of ritualistic structure and to create a sacred space for the person to navigate their challenges. Nevertheless, some of our apprentice students have been exploring in the clinical realm by integrating additional points into the Ghost Points treatment protocol.

Here are a number of examples of some points you could add:

You can generally add additional *Jing*/Well points or any of the Windows to the Sky points, especially in the First Trinity because these points open the orifices (windows) and allow the person to see differently: Lung 3, Bladder 10, Stomach 9, and Large Intestine 18. Or Kidney 1, located on the bottom of the foot, is useful for stabilizing the temperament and the *Shen*/Spirit.

If the person has Heat in the Blood symptoms, you may wish to add points to clear that, such as Spleen 10, Stomach 9, and Bladder 40.

You can also add any points for tonifying qi and blood to build Postnatal qi (qi that is created by nourishment through breathing and eating). You may want to strengthen their Spleen and Postnatal qi, using Spleen 6 or Stomach 42. Or you may want to add Bladder 43 or Bladder 17 to generate more blood and regulate the blood.

If the person is having a hard time telling their story and needs to speak (as we said earlier, it's important that the "heart needs to speak"), you can add a Triple Heater point, like Triple Heater 2 (the Water point in Fire) to help enhance the communication between Fire and Water.

For mental illnesses that seem to be affecting the brain, you can add points that help allow things to come out of the brain, such as Gall Bladder 13 or Gall Bladder 39 to clear the marrow.

For more excessive wind conditions, you can add additional wind points, like Gallbladder 20 (major point along Yang Wei Mai), Gallbladder 31, Bladder 12, Small Intestine 12, or Bladder 10, which is also a pillow (Celestial Pillow) and is nicely paired with Du 16 (Ghost Pillow). Du 17 (as a doorway to the brain, which is often contraindicated for needling) or Du 19 (as a substitute for Du 17) release pathogens from the head and help with poor vision or eye pain.

For phlegm in the nasal passages, you can add Small Intestine 18 as the Sinew Meridian meeting point. We often use this point to "open the orifices," with a "vaporizing phlegm" technique, which uses an Alchemical approach to eliminating phlegm.

If someone is very cold, you can add moxibustion to Bladder 48 (the Yang Shield) to bring up the yang energy and warm the person.

NOTE: There are no Wood ghost points because the ghosts are seeking reincarnation and rebirth, which is what the Wood Element represents. Therefore, when incorporating Wood points, we do not recommend doing them with the Ghost Point method.

Following Up: After a Thirteen Ghost Points Treatment...

The freedom a person feels after a Ghost Points treatment can be hugely transformative or take some time to unfold. However, the treatment is not truly completed until the follow-up treatment is done.

The follow-up treatment plays a crucial role in assisting individuals in rebuilding and reconnecting with their authentic selves. This is a tangible way for a person to discern the contrast between their state before and after treatment. This contrast often manifests as the distinction between the feeling of having no choice of how to live one's life, and the new feeling of true freedom.

After we clear away the blocks and the ghosts, it's really important that a person gets treatment to help them find their authentic selves.

In Chinese Medicine, the Five Elemental energies describe the different types of people in the world. A person might be a Wood type—assertive and efficient. Or they might be a Fire type—outgoing and shy at the same time. An Earth type is very balanced, social, and thoughtful. A Metal type is somewhat introverted but values sincere connection with people. A Water person is all about intensity of movement followed by periods of rest and relaxation.

One of the things we find most helpful when working with people who've struggled very deeply in life is to help them find themselves through understanding their Elemental type and getting treatments that enforce that. There are points on the body that say to a person, "Be you. Be more you." Imagine getting that kind of treatment when all your life you've been told to be someone you're not. It's exactly what you need when you're trying to return to authenticity.

It's also important to make sure that the person's energy is flowing. Some people have Chaotic Energy even after getting rid of their ghosts and blocks. This makes anyone feel pretty crummy. So it's important in the follow-up work to check to make sure all their energy is flowing in their bodies.

Finally, we believe that there's more to life than just getting by and surviving. We always want everyone to achieve their highest potential and fly free in their lives. To be able to fly means that a person is living authentically to the max. They're truly manifesting themselves and all they have to offer to the world. For people ready to do this, we work with what's called "The Nine Stages of Alchemy." These Alchemical stages can be worked through over many years as an evolutionary path for those wishing to become Alchemists. Daoist Alchemists in China have practiced this type of Alchemy for many centuries. Engaging with this approach can guide individuals toward a more complete, confident, and fearless understanding of their existence. We call it learning to really fly in your life. For more information about the Nine Stages of Alchemy, we recommend checking out another one of our books, *Through the Mystery Gate.*

First, seek to find an ultimate state in which you are centered and empty of conscious intention. When the internal and external qi combine in a unified flow, one may take his proper place between heaven and earth, embracing the Yin and the Yang.

—Sun Lutang[21]

[21] Sun Lutang, A *Study of Taijiquan*, trans. Tim Cartell (Berkeley, California: North Atlantic Books, 2003) 73.

Chapter Nine: Conclusion

We like to look at the Thirteen Ghost points as more than a set of points or a protocol, but rather as an experiential container for a transformational opportunity. While it was traditionally used for mental illness and possession, we have found that it is useful for most people we treat who have experienced mild to severe trauma. We like to say it addresses all the ways that trauma and negativity affect a person. It's hard to be alive on this planet without having experienced some trauma and negativity on our path that have changed us in some way, shape, or form, though we believe physical and emotional trauma really has no hierarchy, and everyone experiences pain differently.

By taking this spiritual approach to the Thirteen Ghost points, we're able to see the value they have beyond being able to heal extreme cases of illness. They also address the issues of "regular people," who most modern doctors might not give much attention to. Many people have emotional patterns that are uncomfortable but they may have no way to understand how to shift them. This is the magic, awe, and gentle beauty of this approach.

As a container, the magic of the Thirteen Ghost Points treatment is not in adding more points (though you can if you are inspired to do so), but in ritualistically doing the same points with each person and allowing time and space to open up for that person to find their way. As the treatment creates a safe space for honesty and emotional freedom, it becomes the Alchemical cauldron for transformation and even transmutational change.

An essential aspect of mastering the Ghost Points involves knowing when to insert yourself into the treatment and when to remain an observant guide. It's equally vital to stay in the room with the person, even after the needles are inserted, as they might need time to process the experience with your presence. Regardless of your preference for needles or our energetic (non-needle) approach, the crucial factor is to proceed patiently, allowing space for whatever needs to surface or manifest for the client. We've encountered clients who have told the stories of undergoing a Ghost Points session with other practitioners who left them alone in the room, which can be an emotionally unsettling experience.

The Daoist Alchemists believed that our spirit is perfect. It cannot be harmed or damaged. They used the analogy of Alchemy, the ancient pursuit of turning base minerals into gold, to describe their pursuit and understanding of immortality. Our spirit is like gold. Even after being buried in the ground for thousands of years it comes out untarnished and undamaged. It is incorruptible. Silver and other base minerals, on the other hand, are like our bodies. They are tarnishable and they do degrade over time.

The practice of Alchemy in a human being is the self-led pursuit of the perfection of the spirit within. Through a practice of internal cultivation, a person can undergo a series of powerful Alchemical transformations. Through these transformations, it is believed the Alchemist can become physically immortal and have the ability to fly and transcend time and space.

We feel blessed to be able to offer this work to the world as a new technology for healing trauma and negativity in each of us.

Whether you come to this work for your own healing or as a practitioner wanting to offer more to your clients, learning the Ghost Points always starts with your own self-cultivation. You must first put yourself in this cauldron of change before bringing someone else into it.

This is our experience with these points, and we imagine you will find your own way to engage them. For us it's not only about the points or even the way we do the treatment, but about the role of the practitioner as a conduit for love and hope. We train ourselves to show up with 100% presence and acceptance of all that is. We offer this to our clients with loving kindness. We build a foundation of trust using the points as the vehicle for change.

We offer this approach to you, our readers, and hope this guide is helpful for all those who may need it.

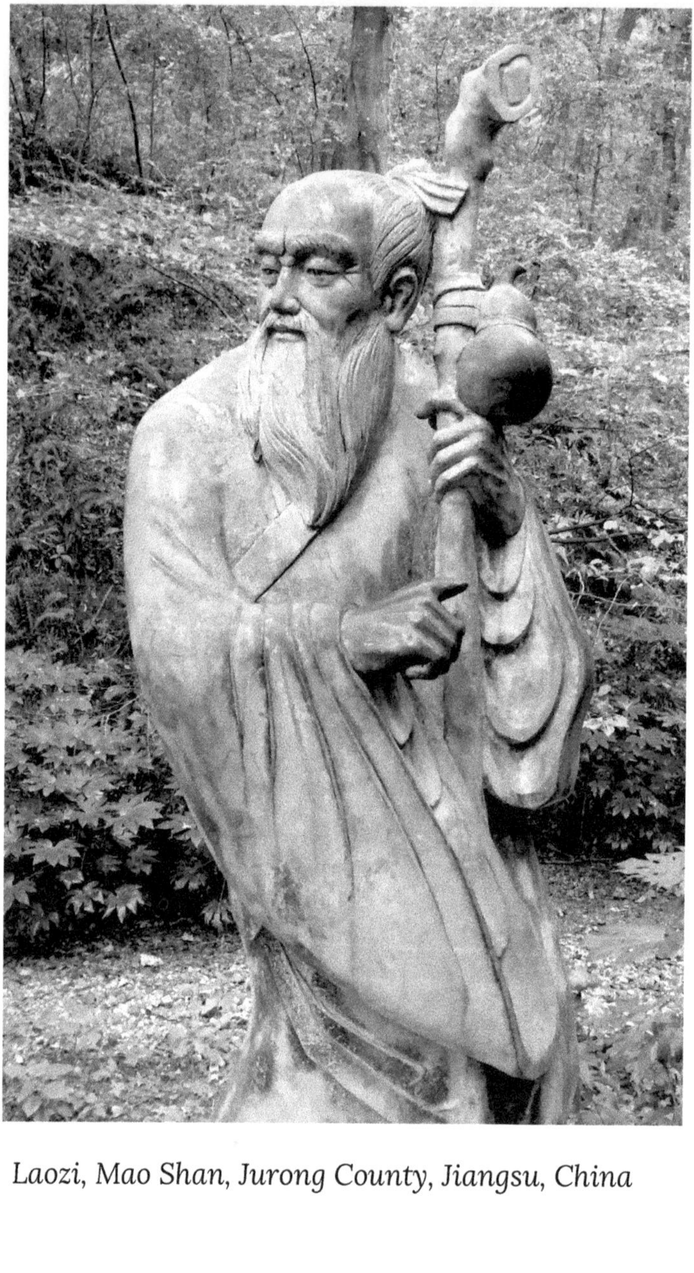

Laozi, Mao Shan, Jurong County, Jiangsu, China

Appendix: Additional Ling Shu Alchemy Treatments

We incorporate several treatments similar to the Thirteen Ghost Points in our Alchemical Chinese Medicine practice. We call these *Ling Shu* treatments, which means spiritual pivot. At the Alchemy Healing Center we often do these *Ling Shu* treatments with new clients to facilitate their return to their authentic selves. These treatments are mostly done with no time restraints and the idea that a huge spiritual pivot or transformation may occur as a result.

The treatment's goal is to reestablish a person's true qi. The result of the treatment is a sense of feeling lighter, like a heavy weight has been lifted away. In this appendix, we will cover the treatments that are pertinent to this book; however, not all treatments are included here. For a complete list, you can visit: AlchemyHealingCenter.com/treatments.

Here is a summary of each treatment type. Each one merits an entire book of its own. That's how important we feel them to be in a self-cultivator's path.

Appendix 1 – The Nine Heart Pains

The Nine Heart Pains Treatment is a treatment we often do after the Thirteen Ghost Points treatment has had time to marinate, usually for at least six months, although it depends on each person's situation. The Nine Heart Pains Treatment is helpful for addictions and a life-long sense of loneliness, isolation, or self-hatred. We also named this "The Loving Yourself" treatment.

Heart pain is an intrinsic component of life. We experience heart pain when a person hurts our feelings or when our dreams cannot be fulfilled. Perhaps it's the pain of not being able to fulfill a career vision. Or perhaps it's the pain of not being wealthy or prosperous. The Nine Palaces of Chinese Medicine relate to the Nine areas of our life that we want to be working properly, and it can be a huge source of heart pain when they are not.

The Nine Palaces Are:

- Career/Knowledge
- Love/Relationship
- Health/Wellness
- Wealth (having enough)/Abundance
- Home (a sense of belonging)
- Adventure/Travel
- Children/Creativity
- Wisdom
- Prosperity (having more than enough)/Charity

Whenever one of these palaces in your life is majorly struggling, you will often experience and accumulate heart pain. The pain of failed relationships and a sense of not belonging or loneliness are two of the most common heart pains.

The Chinese believe that heart pain is unavoidable. In fact, one of the twelve meridians of the body is called the "heart protector." One of its major functions is to heal heart pain.

Heart Pain treatments are used in the following situations:

- When you are trying to overcome an addiction.
- When you have trouble with self-esteem, self-loathing, or an inability to love yourself.
- When you've never felt "at home" in your life.

Appendix 2 - Internal Dragons (IDs)

The Internal Dragons (a.k.a. Internal Devils) ID's Treatment was made popular by the Five Element Chinese Medicine tradition and is taught at Five Element acupuncture schools as a core part of the curriculum. It includes seven points that when activated in a treatment act like keys that open the combination locks on the heart, releasing whatever has a hold on the person.

When a person has had emotional trauma, over time they can build a wall all around their heart. They can become so blocked inside themselves that they can't even access their own heart. It's as if the person has a layer of cellophane wrapped around the heart, and no one can get in and the person can't get out. Trauma or long-term emotional pain can sometimes have such a damaging effect that the person gets lost. We call this an "Internal Heart Block."

According to Chinese Medicine, the heart has a void inside it where our emotions, spirit, and qi can move freely, via the blood. But when the heart is blocked, all of that gets stuck and nothing can move freely. This is how the true aspects of a person can become trapped and lost. If this happens, they cannot proceed with Alchemy. There's no way to move forward if their heart is not under their own control. Another possible reason for this kind of block can be that something else has set up residence in the heart so that the person's spirit is no longer in control of their being.

If the person suspects some kind of entity possession, we don't even need to fully understand the nature of that block, but only to recognize that the person's blocked heart must be released before proceeding with Alchemy.

You can't practice Alchemy if you have a roommate in your heart trying to manifest some other curriculum that is not your own.

The IDs treatment is helpful in the following situations:

- When you feel like you are inaccessible to yourself and/or to others.
- When nothing you try has seemed to help.
- When you feel walled off from the world.
- If you've never felt the same after a traumatic event.
- If you've never felt the same after a long-term emotional upset.

What does an Internal Heart Block feel like? You may feel like you are not at home in your own body. You may behave and function normally, but you feel vacant or vacuous feeling inside. Or sometimes you might feel too intense inside, like you're buzzing. We all have an inherent sense of when something is "off" with a person's spirit. Our eyes are the windows to the soul and since Internal Heart Blocks are caused by deep, soul-level pain, we can easily see this pain in a person's eyes.

While the ID's protocol is well known in the Five Element Chinese Medicine tradition, we approach the ID's treatment in a similar way to treating with the Thirteen Ghost Points. We act as Alchemical Facilitators and offer our clients long sessions—generally four to six hours—to give the time needed to shift blocks that may have been present for many years.

Appendix 3 - External Dragons (EDs)

The External Dragons (a.k.a. External Devils) ED's treatment was made popular by the Five Element Chinese Medicine tradition and is taught at Five Element acupuncture schools as a core part of the curriculum. It includes seven points that when activated in a treatment can release a Will Block, like unlocking a combination lock, releasing whatever has a hold on the person.

If you've been subjugated to another person's will for a long period of time, especially as a child or in an abusive relationship, your Will can become blocked. In that case you can't move forward in your life in any way. You may try, but the forces of your Will cannot be summoned to help you take the next steps.

When a person is unable to move forward in life, no matter how hard they try, they most likely have a Blocked Will. The Chinese believe your Will, meaning the will to survive and take action, is housed in the Kidneys. And it's the Kidneys' job to help you know how to do what you need to do. A person may be completely accessible to their own heart, and they may even have many good ideas of things they want to do, but movement forward in life still somehow seems impossible. We generally recommend the Will Block treatment in the following situations:

- When you have a good sense of what you want to accomplish but you are unable to do it.

- When you feel like you can't get anything done in your life.
- When someone in your life has blocked you from doing what you want and need to do over a long period of time, such as your parents.

This type of block is somewhat uncommon in societies that encourage children to determine their own future, the way it is in the United States where children are often encouraged to choose their own careers. It's more common with people who grow up in more oppressive societal situations or in cultures where children are expected to follow in their parents' footsteps.

While the ED's protocol is well known in the Five Element Chinese Medicine tradition, we approach the ED's treatment in a similar way to treating with the Thirteen Ghost Points. We act as Alchemical Facilitators and offer our clients long sessions—generally four to six hours—to give the time needed to shift blocks that may have been present for many years.

Appendix 4 - Chaotic Energy

When working with a new client or one who hasn't been in for a while, one of the first things we do is to check for Chaotic Energy (a.k.a. Agressive Energy) and whether their energy is flowing freely in the person's energy meridians. Sometimes there are blocks within the meridians that cause various symptoms.

Blocks can be caused by negative emotions or by physical injuries. But often in this chaotic world we are living in, full of 24-hour media bombardment, our energy might not be flowing because it has also become chaotic.

Usually when we tell clients that their energy has become chaotic, they agree wholeheartedly. This is why Leta coined the term "Chaotic Energy" many years ago. Clients with Chaotic Energy often feel like life is out of control. They may feel stressed or anxious or even paranoid. They may have bizarre or unusual physical symptoms that doctors can't really diagnose as an illness (yet). Generally speaking, they just don't feel like themselves. And if you asked any of their family members about it, they might say that their loved one just seems off.

Chaotic Energy often causes the energy flow in your body's merdians to get stuck, sometimes in more than one place. You basically cannot be yourself when this is happening.

The good news is, there is a solution! Chinese Medicine can clear the Chaotic Energy and bring good energy flow back to your body. We typically treat Chaotic Energy at the beginning of most of our Alchemy sessions to ensure that we start off with optimal energy flow in the meridians.

This has become such an important part of our clients' healthcare regime, that we have created a class on Chaotic

Energy that is available at the Alchemy Learning Center (AlchemyLearningCenter.com).

While the Chaotic Energy protocol is well known in the Five Element Chinese Medicine tradition as "Aggressive Energy," we approach this method as Alchemical Facilitators, using non-needle methods of treatment.

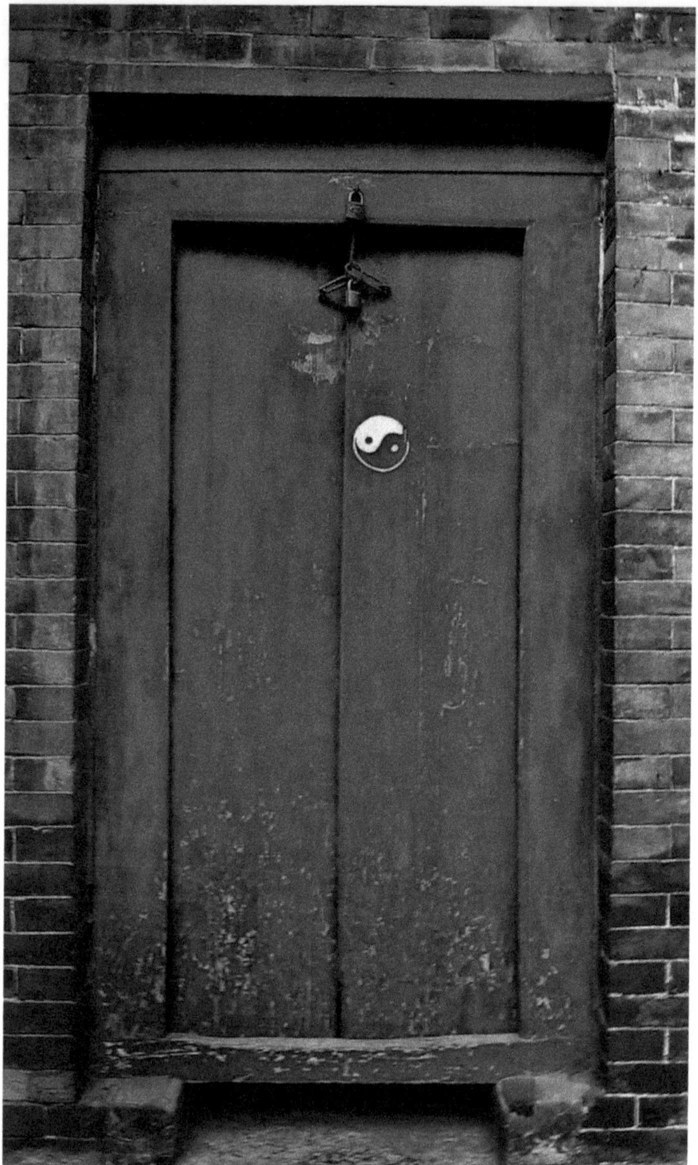

Sun SiMiao's Door at his Home

In 2010, Leta travelled with Master Jeffrey Yuen to the home of Sun SiMiao on Yaowang Mountain in Hunan Province, China. She was profoundly moved by the visit to Yaowang Temple at the mountain's peak, where Daoist monks currently reside.

The simple wooden door in this picture served as the entryway to the monks' quarters. On this battered, scratched, yet beautfiul red door was a Yin-Yang symbol, placed on its side, sitting off-centered. Years later, Jaye found this photograph, restored it to a beautuful image and asked Leta what the sideways Yin-Yang symbol meant. Leta had not noticed or realized it was placed sideways. Curious, she asked Master Yuen about the meaning behind this unusual orientation of the symbol. He explained that when placed on its side, the Yin-Yang symbol represents Alchemy.

This door and its symbol have become the inspiration for so much in our lives, including the Alchemy Healing Center in Northampton, MA, established in 2018. The center features this same magical symbol placed on every door, each painted in the same rich red color. In this way, Leta and all the practitioners at the center are inspired and reminded daily of the legacy of Sun SiMiao.

This amazing, mysterious, and wondrous door has truly opened us up to the world of Alchemy and so much more. Our heartfelt grattitude and desire to understand the mysteries and wonders of the past move us forward to live fully in each and every present moment.

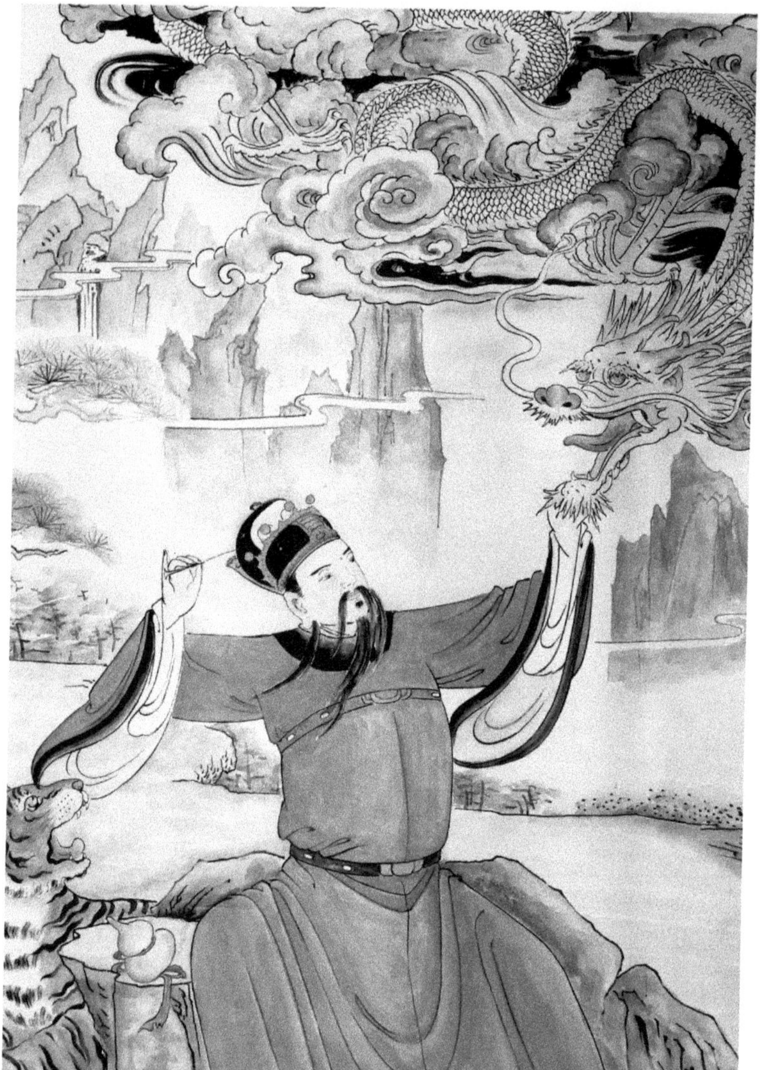

Sun SiMiao Mural

In 2018, Leta and Jaye travelled with Master Jeffrey Yuen to Western China and Tibet. In DunHuang, they visited a small nunnery where an amazing mural was painted on one of the walls, hidden away in a tiny shrine. Jaye was invited into the shrine by one of the nuns and allowed to take this photogragh. We did not know at the time how inspiring and magical this image would become in our lives. We are in grattitude to those who created and perserved this painting and thus, allowed us to share it with the world.

The mural depicts the legend of Sun SiMiao, who is often depited with a dragon and a tiger. In this photogragh. Sun SiMao is treating a dragon's infected mouth. Legend says Sun SiMiao healed both the tiger and the dragon, and the animals repaid his kindness later in life.

Suggested Reading List

After the Ecstasy, the Laundry: How the Heart Grows Wise on the Spiritual Path by Jack Kornfield. Publisher: Bantam, 2001.

As You Thinketh by James Allen. Publisher: Top of the Mountain Publishing, 1989.

Ask and It Is Given: Learning to Manifest Your Desires by Esther and Jerry Hicks. Publisher: Hay House, 2007.

Blessings, Wisdom, and Hurt by Gregg Braden. Publisher: Hay House, 2005.

Change Your Thoughts, Change Your Life by Wayne Dyer. Publisher: Hay House, 2009.

Cultivating Stillness: A Taoist Manual for Transforming Body and Mind by Eva Wong. Publisher: Shambhala, 2012.

Healing Anxiety: A Tibetan Medicine Guide to Healing Anxiety, Stress and PTSD by Mary Friedman-Ryan. Publisher: Born Perfect, 2016.

Lao Tzu: Tao Te Ching: A Book About the Way and the Power of the Way by Ursula K. Le Guin. Publisher: Shambhala, 2019.

Life and Teaching of The Masters of The Far East *by Baird T. Spalding.* Publisher: DeVorss & Company, 1986.

Matrix Energetics: The Science and Art of Transformation by Richard Bartlett. Publisher: Atria Books/ Beyond Words, 2009.

Plant Spirit Medicine: A Journey into the Healing Wisdom of Plants by Eliot Cowan. Publisher: Sounds True, 2014.

Qi Gong for Total Wellness for Total Wellness by Dr. Baolin Wu and Jessica Eckstein. Publisher: St. Martin's Griffin, 2006.

Rooted in Spirit by Claude Larre. Publisher: Barrytown/Station Hill Press, Inc., 1995.

Sastun: One Woman's Apprenticeship with a Maya Healer and Their Efforts to Save the Vani by Rosita Arvigo. Publisher: HarperOne, 1995.

Secrets of the Lost Mode of Prayer: The Hidden Power of Beauty, Blessing, Wisdom, and Hurt by Gregg Braden. Hay House, 2016.

Tales of the Taoist Immortals by Eva Wong. Publisher: Shambhala, 2001.

The Alchemist: A Fable About Following Your Dream, 25th Anniversary Edition by Paulo Coelho. Publisher: HarperOne, 2014.

The Cosmic Serpent: DNA and the Origins of Knowledge by Jeremy Narby. Publisher: Jeremy P. Tarcher/Putnam, 1999.

The Diamond in Your Pocket: Discovering Your True Radiance by Gangaji. Publisher: Sounds True, 2007.

The Disappearance of the Universe by Gary R. Renard. Publisher: Hay House, 2004.

The Master Key System by Charles F. Haanel. Publisher: Filiquarian Publishing, LLC., 2006.

The Power of Now: A Guide to Spiritual Enlightenment by Eckhart Tolle. Publisher: New World Library, 2004.

The Power of Vulnerability: Teachings of Authenticity, Connection, and Courage by Brené Brown. Publisher: Sounds True, 2013.

The Science of Being Well by Wallace D. Wattles. Publisher: Wilder Publications, 2008.

The Secret of the Golden Flower: A Chinese Book of Life translated by Richard Wilhelm. Publisher: Houghton Mifflin Harcourt Publishing Company, 1970.

The Secret Teachings of Plants: The Intelligence of the Heart in the Direct Perception of Nature by Stephen Harrod Buhner. Publisher: Bear Company, 2004.

A Study of Taijiquan by Sun Lutang. Publisher: Blue Snake Books, 2003.

The Tao of Healing: Meditations for Body and Spirit by Haven Trevino. Publisher: New World Library, 1999.

The Wandering Taoist by Ming-Dao Deng. Publisher: HarperCollins, 1986.

The World Is a Waiting Lover: Desire and the Quest for the Beloved by Trebbe Johnson. Publisher: New World Library, 2005.

More from the Authors

Through the Mytery Gate: A Daoist Alchemy Self-Discovery Journey by Leta Herman and Jaye McElroy. Publisher: Born Perfect Ink, 2021.

The Big Little Gua Sha Book: Learning (and Loving) the Ancient Healing Art of Gua Sha by Leta Herman and Jaye McElroy. Publisher: Born Perfect Ink, 2016.

Connecting Your Circle: How the Five Elements Can Help You Be a More Authentic You by Leta Herman and Jaye McElroy. Publisher: Born Perfect Ink, 2014.

The Energy of Love: Applying the Five Elements to Turn Attraction into True Connection by Leta Herman and Jaye McElroy. Publisher: Llewellyn Publications, 2014.

Authenticity is the idea that you are becoming more of everything. That's being truth. Truth is the ability to be all things rather than this thing and not that thing... The idea of Alchemy is that we're constantly trying to separate the pure and turbid, and that purification is the refinement. Purification is inclusion. It's not separation because everything is divine and comes from the divine.

— Jeffrey Yuen[22]

---

[22] Jeffrey Yuen, *Aspects of Chinese Shamanic Practices (from a Chinese Medical & Daoist Perspective), Weekend 2: Sacred Space & the Role of Rituals*, International Tai Chi Institute, New York, NY, March 9-10, 2024.